Delicious Low-Carb Dishes for Newbies

Ravi .S Shah

Delicious Low-Carb Dishes for Newbies : Mouth-Watering Recipes for Starting a Low-Carb Lifestyle Easily and Happily

<u>***Funny helpful tips:***</u>

Maintain clear documentation; it's crucial for audits and compliance.

Stay informed about industry trends; being ahead of the curve gives a competitive edge.

<u>Life advices:</u>

Stay informed about potential allergens; understanding them can prevent adverse reactions.

Your impact is immeasurable; strive to make a positive difference in every interaction.

Introduction

This is a practical guide that introduces readers to the concept of a clean ketogenic diet.

The book provides a 14-day clean keto meal plan, ensuring that individuals can get started with this specific dietary approach easily.

The meal plan is divided into various categories, ensuring that readers have a diverse range of options to choose from. These categories include breakfast, snacks and sides, soups and salads, poultry and seafood, pork and beef, desserts, and sauces and keto staples.

Each section of the meal plan is designed to cater to different tastes and preferences while adhering to the principles of the clean ketogenic diet. Whether someone is looking for a hearty breakfast, a satisfying snack, or a delightful dessert, this book offers a variety of recipes to suit their needs.

By following the provided meal plan and recipes, readers can embark on their clean ketogenic diet journey with confidence, knowing that they have access to delicious and nutritionally balanced meals for a successful and sustainable ketogenic lifestyle.

Contents

The Clean Ketogenic Diet Solution

Welcome to the world of clean keto eating. In this chapter, we start with the fundamentals: what a "clean" ketogenic diet is, how it works, and what its benefits are to you. Not only will you learn what to eat, but I also explain what macronutrients are and how to determine your body's individual needs. By the end of this chapter, you'll have a road map so you can get started on your clean keto journey.

How the Keto Diet Works

There are three types of macronutrients that we consume in the foods we eat: carbohydrates (carbs), fat, and protein. Traditionally, our bodies burn glucose (also called blood sugar) for energy. Glucose enters your bloodstream via the foods you eat (carbohydrates) and is your body's main source of energy.

The ketogenic diet is a low-carb, high-fat, moderate-protein diet. When drastically reducing carbs and instead increasing fats in your diet, while also consuming lean proteins, your body breaks down the fat into ketones instead of burning glucose for energy. In essence, ketones, which are chemicals made in the liver from the breakdown of fats, serve as alternative fuel for your body when glucose is in short supply. When this happens, your body has reached the state of ketosis, when it burns ketones instead of glucose for energy, which is the main goal of the keto diet. The state of ketosis, when paired with exercise, can accelerate weight loss and meeting body composition goals as well as increase energy levels, among other benefits.

The types of foods we put into our bodies are crucially important to the keto diet experience. When following keto, many people make the mistake of thinking it is okay to eat as much cheese, bacon, and butter as they like. While this is okay on occasion, it should not be the norm. Following a clean keto diet (consuming healthy carbs, healthy fats, and lean proteins) is the best way to do your body good on the keto diet. You should also consume vegetables and lower-sugar fruits not only for their nutritional benefits but also for the fiber they provide. Vegetables and lower-sugar fruits should be the main source of carbohydrates while on the keto diet.

"Clean Keto" versus "Dirty Keto"

One of the biggest perks of the keto diet is the flexibility of what you can eat with every meal. With so much freedom of choice, some keto dieters fall into a trap of eating heavily processed foods that are technically allowed on the keto diet but are full of added oils, sugar, and salt (such as deli meats, proteins with high fat content, and keto "snacks" or bars).

While this "dirty keto" or "lazy keto" diet (which relies heavily on greasy proteins and keto-friendly convenience foods that are heavily processed)works for some, it is definitely not for everyone.

To ensure good health for the short and longterm, it's important to embrace a clean eating lifestyle that emphasizes wholesome, nutrient-dense foods such as fresh fruits, vegetables, plant-based proteins, and high-quality meat and seafood.

This extra-healthy version of the keto diet does not allow grains and starches, including corn, rice, wheat and cereal products, or sugar. Instead, most carbohydrates should be obtained from vegetables and fruit.

This fusion of clean eating and the keto diet is what we call "clean keto." In the following pages, you will learn the principles of eating clean keto so you can achieve your own personal health goals, and I share easy recipes and meal plans to help get you there.

CLEAN KETO BENEFITS

A clean eating approach to the keto diet offers several health benefits over the "dirty" keto approach. Here's how it works:

→ Lower blood pressure: Eliminating processed foods that are high in added oils, sodium, or sugar can lower blood pressure.

→ Weight loss: Clean keto (eating real food and keeping the macronutrients within guidelines) may help you lose weight faster.

→ Strengthened immunity: Fueling the body with plenty of fresh vegetables, fruits, lean protein, and healthy fats helps protect the body from disease.

→ Powerful anti-inflammatory benefits: Studies have shown that the keto diet is anti-inflammatory. Inflammation can cause arthritic pain and has been linked to Alzheimer's disease, asthma, cancer, diabetes, and heart disease. Following the keto diet may aid in reducing inflammation when the body reaches a state of ketosis.

→ Increased focus and energy: When the body starts burning ketones instead of glucose, and blood sugar stabilizes, brain function may improve, and energy levels may become more stable.

Clean Keto Fundamentals

When beginning a clean keto diet, you'll need to make some changes in how you grocery shop and menu plan. To help, this book contains 75 recipes and 2 weekly meal plans, as well as tips on how to stay in ketosis (see here). Additionally, keeping the following overarching guidelines top of mind will help you stick to your clean eating plan, which will also increase your energy and keep you feeling satisfied, helping you to avoid any "dirty eating" traps.

Choose Quality Food

Good quality, nutritious food that's as close to its natural state as possible (that is, unprocessed) is more likely to deliver the macronutrients your body needs. Choosing organic produce is recommended because it has not been treated with chemicals or preservatives and is pesticide-free. Organic, grass-fed meat and poultry are also recommended because they don't contain any antibiotics or hormones. However, both choices often cost slightly more than nonorganic. If funds don't allow for the extra expense, just choose the highest quality of fresh food you can reasonably afford. You'll still find success on clean keto.

Mind Your Sugar and Salt Intake

Sugar is a carbohydrate that turns into glucose, and glucose is what the body turns to for energy. (Your body will burn glucose before it burns fat.) Eating too much sugar can cause weight gain and raise blood sugar levels, which can put you at a risk for diabetes.

Rather than using sugar, turn to natural sweeteners like monk fruit, stevia, or erythritol. Each of these natural sweeteners is calorie-free and does not affect blood sugar. Fruit contains natural sugars and is okay to consume as long as you are staying in the 5% carbohydrate range (see here). I list the best fruits to consume in the "Foods to Eat and Avoid on the Clean Keto Diet" section on here.

When eliminating processed foods from your diet, you may find that your sodium levels drop. That is because processed foods contain high quantities of salt. It may sound odd, but you might need to increase your salt intake on keto, contradicting the general recommendation of limiting salt. Signs you may not be getting enough sodium in your diet are muscle cramps or spasms, fatigue, irritability, nausea, and confusion.

Avoid Processed Foods

Avoid processed foods such as grains, starches, refined oils, processed meats, and artificial sweeteners (aspartame, sucralose, and saccharin) on the keto diet. Processed foods are often high in sodium, and processed meats typically contain nitrates, which are used to extend the shelf life of bacon and lunch meats, for example.

High levels of sodium and nitrates can increase the risk of heart disease and contribute to inflammation. Inflammation may cause fatigue, feelings of general unwellness, and even fever. By simply removing processed foods from your diet, you may notice increased energy and a feeling of well-being. The long-term benefits of eliminating processed foods include reducing the risk of heart disease, obesity, arthritis, Alzheimer's, and more.

Eat the Rainbow

The body needs vitamins and minerals to nourish and maintain good health. Eating a variety of whole foods aids in providing your body those vitamins and minerals. The five micronutrients that play roles in maintaining a healthy body are vitamin B_6, vitamin C, vitamin E, magnesium, and zinc. Consuming fruits and vegetables of different colors daily, or "eating the rainbow," is a great way to increases your intake of a variety of vitamins and nutrients.

Some micronutrient-rich vegetables that are keto-friendly include spinach; green and purple cabbage; broccoli; red, green, and yellow bell peppers; kale; and zucchini. Fruits that all fit the micronutrient guidelines for keto include blackberries, blueberries, strawberries, and tomatoes.

Understanding the Keto Ratio

Two fundamentals to success with the keto diet are (1) an understanding of what macronutrients (or "macros") are (carbohydrates, fat, and protein), and (2) staying in ketosis.

For the keto diet to work optimally, a certain ratio of fat, carbohydrates, and proteins need to be maintained. Because each body is different, I recommend using an app or website like Carb Manager (see here) to help you easily calculate and track what your body needs in terms of daily calories and macros.

Each macro plays an important part in the keto diet so it's imperative to reach daily intake goals. Combining these macros with an array of healthy foods that don't contain added oil, sugar, or salt is key to success.

Carbohydrates: 5%

Carbohydrates contain about 4 calories per gram and should make up 5% of your daily caloric intake on the keto diet. Most of your carbohydrates should come from keto-friendly fruits and vegetables, though some carbs will come from dairy products such as Greek yogurt and cheese, as well as nut flours and milks. On the keto diet, net carbs—not total carbs—are the number to track in terms of your daily intake (for most, this number is roughly 20 to 25 grams per day). Net carbs are determined by subtracting the grams of fiber (a type of carb not easily absorbed by the body and therefore not as impactful on blood sugar) and sugar alcohols from grams of total carbs consumed.

Fat: 70%

Healthy fats should make up 70% of the calories you consume daily on the keto diet. Fat is one of the macronutrients that helps keep you satisfied and feeling full longer and contains roughly 9 calories per gram. Foods like avocados, nuts, and olives are examples of high-fat foods with great nutritional benefits. Other foods that contain healthy fats and are often used in keto recipes are flaxseed, chia seed, psyllium husk, and hemp hearts.

Proteins: 25%

Protein contains about 4 calories per gram and should make up 25% of the calories you consume daily on the keto diet. It is important to eat a variety of proteins to help preserve muscle mass during a low-carb diet. Some of the best lean proteins to consume are fish, seafood, lean beef, pork, chicken, and eggs. Be sure to eat a variety of proteins throughout the week for maximum nutritional benefits and to help prevent boredom with meals.

Foods to Embrace

Healthy Fats

- Animal Fats
  + Butter (unsalted)
  + Ghee
  + Lard
  + Mayonnaise
  + Tallow

- Nut Butters
  + Almond butter
  + Cocoa butter
  + Coconut butter

- Unrefined Oils
  + Avocado oil
  + Coconut oil
  + Extra-virgin olive oil
  + Macadamia oil
  + MCT oil

- Other
  + Avocado
  + Coconut milk, full-fat
  + Nuts (almonds, macadamia nuts, pecans walnuts)
  + Olives

- Beef
    + Ground
    + Steak (fillet, flank, rib-eye, skirt)
    + Tenderloin

- Chicken (ground, quarters, thighs, whole)
- Eggs
- Organ Meats
    + Collagen powder
    + Liver
    + Tripe

- Pork
    + Bacon
    + Chops
    + Ground sausage
    + Tenderloin

- Fish and Seafood
    + Salmon
    + Sardines
    + Scallops
    + Sea bass
    + Shrimp
    + Trout
    + Tuna

- Turkey (ground, quarters, slices—precooked, thighs, whole)

Nonstarchy Vegetables

+ Artichokes
+ Asparagus
+ Bok choy
+ Broccoli
+ Brussels sprouts
+ Cabbage
+ Cauliflower
+ Celery
+ Chard
+ Chives
+ Cucumber (English)
+ Eggplant
+ Endive
+ Fennel
+ Garlic
+ Green beans
+ Kale
+ Leeks
+ Lettuce
+ Mushrooms
+ Okra
+ Onions
+ Peppers
+ Radicchio
+ Radishes
+ Rhubarb
+ Spinach
+ Sprouts
+ Tomatoes
+ Water chestnuts
+ Zucchini

Beverages

- Bone broth
- Coffee (no natural sweetener)
- Seltzer/sparkling water (unflavored)
- Tea (unsweetened and not instant)
- Water

Flavorings

- Black pepper (freshly ground)
- Dried herbs and spices
- Fresh herbs
- Lemon
- Lime
- Mustard (Dijon, yellow)
- Pink Himalayan salt
- Vinegars (apple cider, balsamic, and red wine)

Foods to Eat in Moderation

- Dairy (1 cup max per day)

    + Cheese (full-fat)
    + Cream (heavy)
    + Greek yogurt (full-fat, plain)

- Fruits (½ cup max per day)

    + Blackberries
    + Blueberries

+ Raspberries
+ Strawberries

Foods to Avoid

- All grains and starches (bread, cereal, corn, rice, wheat, etc.)
- Artificial sweeteners (Equal, Splenda, Sweet'n Low, etc.)
- Beer, ciders, and sweet wines/liquors
- Energy drinks
- Fruit-based smoothies
- Fruit juice
- Low-fat and diet products containing artificial ingredients/sweeteners
- Margarine
- Most fruits (apples, bananas, oranges, etc.)
- Processed foods
- Refined oils (canola, corn, grape seed, soybean, vegetable)
- Soda/diet soda
- Starchy vegetables (butternut squash, plantains, potatoes, sweet potatoes, etc.)
- Sugar (agave, evaporated cane juice, high fructose corn syrup, honey, maple syrup, powdered sugar, white and brown sugar, etc.)

Staying in Ketosis

Once your body has reached the state of ketosis, it is important to keep it there. There are several ways to tell if you have reached ketosis: urine test strips and blood meters are helpful tools for monitoring ketosis, while some of the physical signs are bad breath, weight loss, decreased hunger, and increased focus and energy.

Many people who reach ketosis experience what's called the "keto flu." The symptoms range from fatigue, irritability, and insomnia to headache and constipation. It is not known why some people experience keto flu, but it's likely a by-product of carb withdrawal or simply the shock of consuming a cleaner diet. These symptoms typically last from just a few days to a week. Take some comfort from knowing that it is a common experience, and you will get over it. If it lingers for longer than a week, you should talk to your doctor before continuing.

If you consume too many carbs after reaching ketosis, your body can fall out of ketosis. To get back into ketosis quickly, try intermittent fasting (see [here](#)) and track your carb intake, making sure to stay within the 5% of net carbs allowed.

Leveraging Intermittent Fasting

Intermittent fasting, abstaining from food or drink for a prescribed amount of time, is a popular eating strategy used to help achieve health and weight loss goals while on the keto diet. While fasting is not a requirement, it is a tool you can use to reach ketosis faster and a helpful strategy for losing weight: when the body is in ketosis, it is burning fat.

Eating fewer meals results in lower caloric intake, and fasting lowers insulin and increases the release of the fat-burning hormone. Short-term fasting may also increase your metabolic rate.

There are many ways to fast. A common approach is a 16-hour period of fasting followed by an 8-hour window of eating. For example, in a 16-hour fast, you would eat your last meal of the day by 5 or 6 p.m., and then not eat again until 10 a.m. the following day.

If fasting is something you're considering, I highly recommend starting out with a 16-hour fast and monitoring how your body reacts to it before increasing the fast window. And, as always, check with your physician before making any major adjustments to your diet.

The Recipes in This Book

In this book, I've provided clean keto diet recipes that can be enjoyed on their own or as part of the meal plans detailed in chapter 2. Each recipe keeps health and ease of use top of mind. To help guide you, each recipe includes labels indicating if it can be made in one pot, has five or fewer ingredients (not including basics such as extra-virgin olive oil, olive oil cooking spray, salt, pepper, and water), is quick to prep (10 minutes or less), or if it can be made in 30 minutes or less.

Dairy-free, vegetarian, or recipes that are "worth the wait" (45 minutes or more) will be labeled as such. Many recipes contain tips for substitutions, variations, or shopping and all include nutritional information to assist in keeping track of macronutrients.

Please note that the recipes in this book were crafted with ingredients from specific brands I use in my own kitchen, which can impact nutritional calculations. I've included the names of those brands when possible, but always read the nutritional labels on any ingredients you use to ensure that your macronutrient needs are met.

CLEAN KETO SWAPS

Adjusting to a clean keto lifestyle is not hard once you understand how to make a few simple ingredient swaps. Some foods that you see on store shelves may seem like they are keto-friendly but are not, so always read the ingredient list on any product you're considering. Here are some basic swaps to get you started:

→ Replace pasta noodles with zucchini noodles.

→ Make <u>Avocado Oil Mayonnaise</u> in place of store-bought mayonnaise.

→ Use unsweetened almond milk in place of cream in beverages.

→ Buy cauliflower flatbreads instead of low-carb flour tortillas.

→ Swap in <u>Cauliflower Fried Rice</u> for regular rice.

→ Use lettuce leaves in place of burger buns.

→ Use natural sweeteners like erythritol, monk fruit, or stevia in place of artificial sweeteners (aspartame, saccharin, etc.).

→ Make low-carb <u>Chia Seed Jam</u> instead of using sugar-free jam, which is likely sweetened with artificial sweeteners.

→ Enjoy plain Greek yogurt with a few berries on top instead of yogurt sweetened with artificial sweeteners.

→ Use coconut aminos in place of soy sauce.

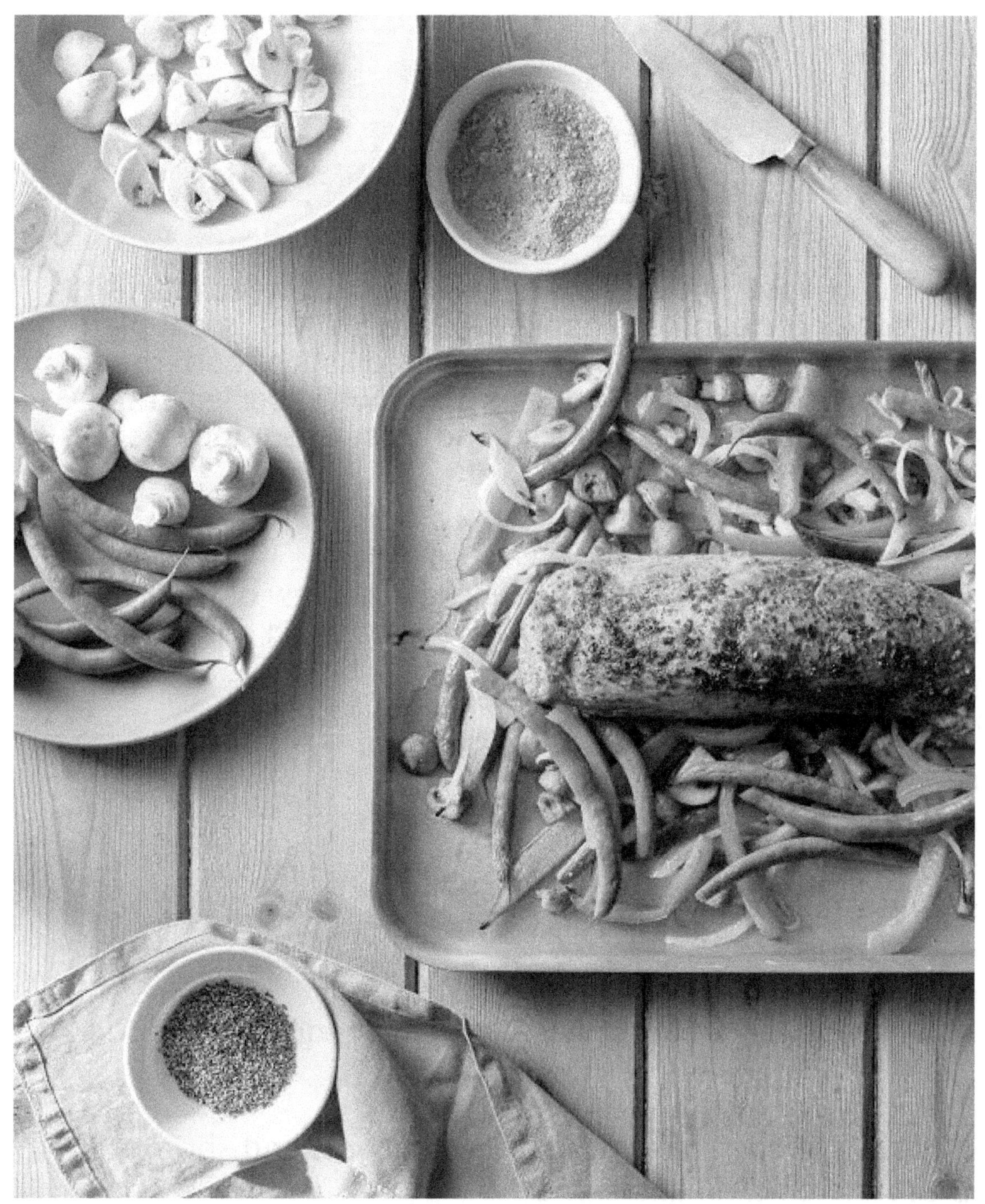

2

14-Day Clean Keto Meal Plan

This chapter focuses on everything you need to start cooking clean keto as well as a two-week meal plan to help you get started. I've provided lists of both the fresh ingredients you should stock up on as well as shelf-stable and freezer staples. You'll also find a list of equipment to have on hand.

Stocking Your Clean Keto Kitchen

To follow a clean keto lifestyle, here are a few of the ingredients and equipment to always have on hand.

Refrigerator and Freezer Staples

- ☐ Almond milk (unsweetened)
- ☐ Berries
- ☐ Broccoli
- ☐ Butternut squash
- ☐ Cabbage
- ☐ Cauliflower
- ☐ Cheese (blue, cream cheese, full-fat cheddar, shredded part-skim mozzarella, and Swiss)
- ☐ Eggs
- ☐ Frozen haddock, salmon fillets, scallops, and shrimp
- ☐ Ground chicken and turkey
- ☐ Ground pork and beef

- ☐ Lemons and limes
- ☐ Mushrooms
- ☐ Onions
- ☐ Pork chops and beef steak
- ☐ Radishes
- ☐ Romaine lettuce
- ☐ Summer squash (green and yellow)
- ☐ Tomatoes
- ☐ Unsalted butter

Pantry Staples

- ☐ Almond flour (be sure to purchase finely ground almond flour)
- ☐ Canned chicken and tuna fish
- ☐ Canned tomatoes
- ☐ Cocoa powder (unsweetened)
- ☐ Coconut flour
- ☐ Natural sweeteners (classic granulated, brown, and powdered; I recommend Lankato Monkfruit and Swerve brands)
- ☐ Nuts (almonds, macadamia nuts, pecans, and walnuts)
- ☐ Olive oil (extra-virgin)
- ☐ Olive oil cooking spray
- ☐ Red hot sauce
- ☐ Salt and black pepper
- ☐ Sugar-free chocolate chips (Lily's brand is excellent)
- ☐ Unsweetened coconut flakes

- ☐ Baking pans (8-by-8-inch and 9-by-13-inch)
- ☐ Baking sheet
- ☐ Cake pans (8-inch round)
- ☐ Cheese grater
- ☐ Knives (chef's and paring, used for chopping and peeling)
- ☐ Mini waffle iron (to make chaffles)
- ☐ Mixing bowls (small, medium, and large)
- ☐ Parchment paper
- ☐ Pizza pan
- ☐ Plastic storage containers with lids
- ☐ Skillets (small and large)
- ☐ Spatulas

14 Days of Clean Keto Meals

Having a simple meal plan is a good way to get into the groove of cooking on a clean keto diet. Plus, by planning meals and snacks ahead of time, you'll be set up to stay on track and avoid temptation.

Because some people experience the "keto flu" (see here) when starting the keto diet, this 14-day meal plan is designed to provide the energy and nutrition needed to adjust to this way of eating. Be sure to stay hydrated, reduce caffeine intake if sleep is troublesome, and avoid strenuous exercise for these first two weeks. Use an app or website, like Carb Manager (see here), to keep close track of macros and be sure to consume the proper ratio of carbohydrates, fats, and proteins (see here).

This meal plan is intended for two people. You can easily scale the recipes down to feed just one person or scale up to feed a family of four. A few of the recipes serve four to six people, and you can enjoy the leftovers at other meals throughout the week or can freeze them for later consumption (for example, leftover Keto Chicken Nuggets and Pulled Pork). If you are cooking for one, you might want to consider substituting a hearty salad, soup, or stir-fry in place of some of the larger meals. If cooking for four people or more, go with a recipe that will yield more per serving while staying within the macros needed.

Week 1 Meal Plan

	Breakfast	Lunch	Dinner	Snack (optional)
Sunday	Chocolate Chip Chaffles and Keto Maple Syrup	Roasted Cauliflower Salad	Homemade Fish Sticks and Creamy Coleslaw	Celery sticks stuffed with cream cheese, sprinkled with everything bagel seasoning
Monday	Leftover Chocolate Chip Chaffles and Keto Maple Syrup	Leftover Homemade Fish Sticks and Creamy Coleslaw	Pulled Pork and Leftover Roasted Cauliflower Salad	Spiced Mug Cake (double recipe)
Tuesday	2 scrambled	Italian Wedding	Leftover Pulled	½ cup berries and

	eggs (each) and Homemade Breakfast Sausage	Soup	Pork in Romaine Lettuce Cups or Cauliflower Tortillas and Creamy Coleslaw	½ cup plain Greek yogurt (each)
Wednesday	Cinnamon Roll Pancakes and Leftover Homemade Breakfast Sausage	Leftover Italian Wedding Soup	Cheesy-Stuffed Chicken with Spicy Sauce	1 hard-boiled egg (each) and Chipotle Ranch Dressing
Thursday	Layered StrawberryChia Pudding	Leftover Italian Wedding Soup	Leftover Cheesy-Stuffed Chicken with Spicy Sauce	Sweet bell pepper and cucumber slices and Leftover Chipotle Ranch Dressing
Friday	Leftover Cinnamon Roll Pancakes and Homemad	Keto Chicken Nuggets and cucumber and	Pork Chops and Cauliflower Fried Rice	Leftover Layered Strawberry Chia Pudding

		tomato salad		
	e Breakfast Sausage			
Saturday	Coffee with heavy cream and ½ cup berries with ½ cup Greek yogurt (each)	Leftover Pork Chops and Cauliflower Fried Rice	Beef and Broccoli Stir-Fry	Keto Hummus and cucumber slices

Week 1 Shopping List

Week 1's shopping list is large because it includes staples as well as ingredients. Check your pantry for items you may already have.

PRODUCE

☐ Berries
• Blackberries, blueberries, raspberries, or strawberries (1 container, your choice)
• Strawberries (1-quart)
☐ Broccoli (1 crown)
☐ Cabbage, green (1 small head)
☐ Cabbage, purple (1 small head)
☐ Cauliflower (3 heads)
☐ Cauliflower, riced (2 cups)
☐ Celery (1 bunch)
☐ Cucumber, English (1)
☐ Garlic cloves (2 heads)

□ Ginger paste (1 tube)
□ Grape tomatoes (1 pint)
□ Jalapeño pepper (1) (optional)
□ Lemons (2)
□ Lime (1)
□ Parsley (1 bunch)
□ Red bell pepper (2)
□ Romaine lettuce (1 head)
□ Sage, fresh (1)
□ Scallions (1 bunch)
□ Thyme, fresh (1 bunch)
□ Yellow onion (2)

DAIRY AND EGGS

□ Almond milk, unsweetened (64 ounces)
□ Butter, unsalted (1 pound)
□ Cream cheese (2 [8-ounce] packages)
□ Cheddar cheese (8 ounces)
□ Crumbly blue cheese (8 ounces)
□ Eggs, large (1 dozen)
□ Feta cheese (8 ounces)
□ Greek yogurt, plain full-fat (8 ounces)
□ Heavy (whipping) cream (16 ounces)
□ Mozzarella cheese, shredded part-skim (8 ounces)
□ Parmesan cheese, grated (8 ounces)
□ Sour cream, full-fat (8 ounces)

MEAT

□ Beef tenderloin (1 pound)
□ Chicken breasts, boneless, skinless (1½ pounds)
□ Cod fish (1 pound)
□ Ground beef, 80/20 (1 pound)
□ Pork, bone in (4 chops)
□ Pork, ground (1 pound)
□ Pork, shoulder roast (4 pounds)
□ Turkey, ground (12 ounces)

PANTRY

□ Almond flour (1 pound)
□ Apple cider vinegar (1 small bottle/16 ounces)
□ Baking powder (1 package/8 ounces)
□ Canned chicken (1 [12.5-ounce] can)
□ Chia seeds (1 small bag/32 ounces)
□ Chicken broth, reduced-sodium, (3 [32-ounce] cartons)
□ Chipotle peppers with adobo sauce (1 can)
□ Chocolate chips, sugar-free (1 bag/8 ounces)
□ Coconut aminos (1 bottle/10 ounces, I use Coconut Secret)
□ Coconut flour (16 ounces)
□ Coffee
□ Gelatin, unflavored (1 box/1 ounce)
□ Hot sauce (1 bottle)
□ Kalamata olives, pitted (1 jar/9½ ounces)
□ Maple-flavored syrup, sugar-free (1 bottle/14 ounces)
□ Mayonnaise, keto-friendly (32 ounces, I like Primal Kitchen brand)
□ Mustard, yellow (8 ounces)

☐ Olive oil, extra-virgin (1 bottle/32 ounces)
☐ Rice vinegar, unseasoned (1 bottle/12 ounces)
☐ Roasted red bell peppers (1 small jar/16 ounces)
☐ Sesame oil (8 ounces)
☐ Sweet chili sauce, sugar-free (1 bottle/12 ounces)
☐ Sweetener, natural sugar-free, granulated, powdered, and brown (1 [48-ounce] package of each)
☐ Pure vanilla extract (1 bottle/2 ounces)
☐ Tahini (8 ounces)

HERBS AND SPICES

☐ Black pepper, freshly ground
☐ Cayenne pepper, ground
☐ Celery seed, whole
☐ Chili powder
☐ Cinnamon, ground
☐ Cloves, ground
☐ Cumin, ground
☐ Everything bagel seasoning
☐ Fennel seeds
☐ Garlic powder
☐ Ginger, ground
☐ Nutmeg, ground
☐ Old Bay seasoning
☐ Onion powder
☐ Red pepper flakes (optional)
☐ Salt
☐ Smoked paprika

	Breakfast	Lunch	Dinner	Snack (optional)
Sunday	Leftover Layered Strawberry Chia Pudding	Leftover Beef and Broccoli Stir-Fry	Keto Cabbage Roll Casserole	¼ cup almonds, macadamia nuts, or pecans (each)
Monday	Coffee with heavy cream and ½ cup fresh berries with ½ cup Greek yogurt (each)	Sweet and Spicy Broccoli Salad	Leftover Keto Cabbage Roll Casserole	Leftover Keto Hummus and cucumber slices
Tuesday	Blueberry Ricotta Crepes	Leftover Sweet and Spicy Broccoli Salad	Leftover Keto Cabbage Roll Casserole	2 ounces Swiss cheese and 2 tomato slices (each)
Wednesday	2 scrambled eggs (each) and Raspberry Muffins	Leftover Sweet and Spicy Broccoli Salad	Sheet Pan Pork Tenderloin with Veggies	Leftover Keto Hummus and cucumber slices
Thursday	Eggs with Goat Cheese	Creamy Chicken	Leftover Sheet Pan	¼ cup almonds,

	and Asparagus	Mushroom Soup	Pork Tenderloin with Veggies	macadamia nuts, or pecans (each)
Friday	1 egg omelet made with Leftover Sheet Pan Pork Tenderloin with Veggies	Leftover Creamy Chicken Mushroom Soup	Maple-Garlic Salmon with Toasted Walnuts	2 ounces Swiss cheese and 2 tomato slices (each)
Saturday	Coffee with heavy cream and Leftover Raspberry Muffins	Leftover Creamy Chicken Mushroom Soup	Leftover Maple-Garlic Salmon with Toasted Walnuts	Chocolate Bark with Walnuts

Week 2 Shopping List

Note that for convenience and to avoid waste, some of the meals served in week 1 are served as leftovers during week 2. You can also freeze leftovers from week 2 to eat later, like Keto Cabbage Roll Casserole or Raspberry Muffins. As you prepare to shop for week 2, be sure to check your pantry and refrigerator for ingredients you already have and won't need to purchase.

PRODUCE

☐ Asparagus (1 bunch)
☐ Bell peppers (1 red, 1 green)
☐ Broccoli (2 crowns)

- ☐ Blueberries (1 pint)
- ☐ Cabbage, green (1 small head)
- ☐ Cauliflower, riced (3 cups)
- ☐ Garlic (1 head)
- ☐ Green beans (8 ounces)
- ☐ Jalapeño pepper (1)
- ☐ Lemon (1)
- ☐ Mushrooms, button (24 ounces)
- ☐ Onions, yellow (2)
- ☐ Parsley (1 bunch)
- ☐ Raspberries (1 pint)
- ☐ Sage leaves (1 bunch)
- ☐ Scallions (1 bunch)
- ☐ Tomato (1)

DAIRY AND EGGS

- ☐ Almond milk, unsweetened (64 ounces)
- ☐ Butter, unsalted (8 ounces)
- ☐ Cheddar cheese, full-fat (8 ounces)
- ☐ Cheese, ricotta, ½ cup
- ☐ Cream cheese, full-fat (10 ounces)
- ☐ Eggs, large (2 dozen)
- ☐ Goat cheese, full-fat (4 ounces)
- ☐ Greek yogurt, plain full-fat (1 [5–6 ounce] container)
- ☐ Parmesan cheese, grated (1 package/8 ounces)
- ☐ Swiss cheese (1 [7-ounce] package)

MEAT

- ☐ Bacon, nitrate- and sugar-free (1 pound)
- ☐ Ground beef, 80/20 (1¼ pounds)
- ☐ Chicken tenders (1 pound)
- ☐ Pork tenderloin (2 pounds)
- ☐ Salmon (4 [4-ounce] fillets)

- ☐ Chicken broth, reduced-sodium (16 ounces)
- ☐ Sugar-free dark chocolate chips (8 ounces)
- ☐ Dijon mustard
- ☐ Nuts
- •Almonds, macadamia nuts, or pecans (1 container, your choice)
- • Walnuts (3.5 ounces/1½ cups)
- ☐ Pasta sauce, low-carb (1 cup)
- ☐ Pure almond extract
- ☐ Sunflower seeds, unsalted (½ cup)

After the Meal Plan

When building future menus, remember to consider the number of peoplewho will be eating with you. I like to scale up the size of a main course, such as Pulled Pork, so that I can repurpose the leftovers for another meal,such as Pulled Pork–Stuffed Mushrooms. Mealtimes are so mucheasier when you can consume leftovers for lunch or dinner the next day or two.

If you find that you are having a hard time consuming enough fat in a day, adding an avocado to a salad or serving it as a side to eggs for breakfast is a good way to boost fats in a heathy way.

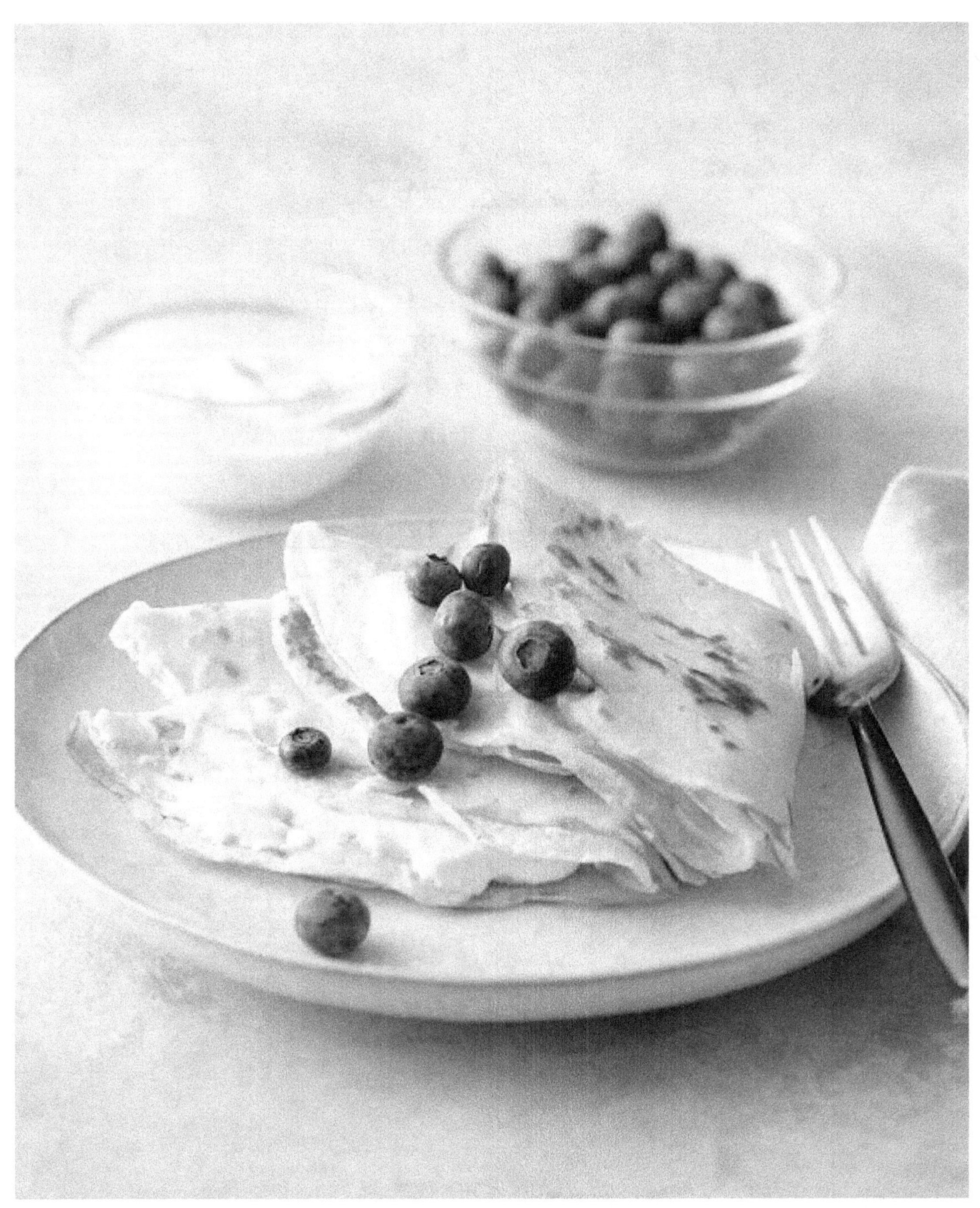

Blueberry Ricotta Crepes

3

Breakfast

Blueberry Ricotta Crepes
Cinnamon Roll Pancakes
Chocolate Chip Chaffles
Raspberry Muffins
Layered Strawberry Chia Pudding
Egg and Sausage Cauliflower Hash
Egg in a Hole Pepper Rings
Mushroom Cheese Omelet
Eggs with Goat Cheese and Asparagus
Loaded Breakfast Bowls
Homemade Breakfast Sausage

Blueberry Ricotta Crepes

SERVES: 4 | Vegetarian
PREP TIME: 10 minutes, plus 10 minutes rest time | COOK TIME: 20 minutes

Don't let the word "crepes" fool you. These thin pancakes are quick, delicious, and versatile. Make these in a blender so the cheese and eggs are thoroughly incorporated, and you end up with a smooth batter. Soften the cream cheese before blending. If needed, warm the cream cheese in the microwave for 10 seconds before using.

FOR THE CREPES

2 ounces full-fat cream cheese, softened

2 large eggs, room temperature

¼ cup unsweetened almond milk

½ teaspoon pure vanilla extract

⅓ cup almond flour

1 tablespoon granulated natural sweetener

Olive oil cooking spray

FOR THE FILLING

½ cup full-fat ricotta cheese

¼ cup powdered natural sweetener

¼ teaspoon pure almond extract

½ cup fresh blueberries

TO MAKE THE CREPES

1. In a blender, combine the cream cheese, eggs, almond milk, vanilla, almond flour, and natural sweetener. Cover with the lid and process until the batter is smooth. Set aside to rest for 10 minutes.

2. Heat a 10-inch skillet over medium heat. Remove the pan from the heat, lightly coat the bottom of the skillet with cooking spray, and return the pan to the heat.

3. Add ¼ cup of the batter to the center of the hot skillet and swirl to spread into a thin layer that reaches the skillet's edges. Cook for 2 minutes or until the edges are cooked and the center looks slightly dry. Flip and cook on the other side for 2 more minutes, or until the crepe is lightly browned.

4. Remove the crepe from the pan and place on a plate lined with parchment paper. Repeat with the remaining batter, placing a piece of parchment paper between each crepe to prevent them from sticking.

TO MAKE THE FILLING

5. In a small bowl, stir together the ricotta cheese, powdered natural sweetener, and almond extract until thoroughly combined.

6. Place a large dollop of the filling in the center of the crepe and spread evenly. Then fold the right side of the crepe just past the middle of the filling. Repeat with the left side.

7. Top each serving with ¼ cup blueberries.

VARIATION: Try using lemon or orange extract in the ricotta filling instead of almond. Raspberries, blackberries, or strawberries can be substituted for the blueberries.

PER SERVING: Calories: 182; Total fat: 14g; Total carbs: 23g; Fiber: 1.5g; Net carbs: 6.5g; Protein: 7g

Cinnamon Roll Pancakes

These pancakes puff up nice and thick, just like the pancakes I remember from my childhood. Coconut flour helps thicken the batter. If you prefer a less sweet pancake, you can omit the granulated natural sweetener. I love to serve these pancakes on the weekend with a side of <u>Homemade Breakfast Sausage</u>.

FOR THE PANCAKES

4 ounces full-fat cream cheese, softened

2 large eggs

½ teaspoon pure vanilla extract

⅓ cup almond flour

2 tablespoons coconut flour

1 tablespoon granulated natural sweetener (optional)

½ tablespoon baking powder

1 teaspoon ground cinnamon

⅛ teaspoon salt

2 tablespoons unsalted butter

FOR THE FROSTING (OPTIONAL)

¼ cup powdered natural sweetener

1 tablespoon unsalted butter, melted

1 tablespoon full-fat cream cheese, softened

1½ teaspoons unsweetened almond milk

⅛ teaspoon pure vanilla extract

TO MAKE THE PANCAKES

1. In a blender, combine the cream cheese, eggs, and vanilla. Cover with the lid and process for 1 minute or until smooth.

2. Add the almond flour, coconut flour, natural sweetener (if using), baking powder, cinnamon, and salt. Cover and process for 1 minute or until smooth. Set the batter aside for 5 minutes to rise slightly and thicken.

3. Meanwhile, heat a large skillet over medium heat until hot. Add 1 teaspoon of the butter and heat until melted and bubbling.

4. Spacing them evenly, spoon 1 tablespoon mounds of batter into the hot skillet, spreading slightly with a spoon. Only put as many mounds of batter as possible without the edges touching. Cook pancakes for 1 minute or until the edges begin to brown and the centers bubble and begin to look slightly dry. Carefully flip the pancakes over and cook for another 30 seconds or until the bottoms are lightly browned. Transfer pancakes to a plate and keep warm. Repeat with any remaining batter.

TO MAKE THE FROSTING (IF USING)

5. In a small bowl, using a wooden spoon, combine the natural sweetener, butter, cream cheese, almond milk, and vanilla until smooth. Drizzle over the top of the pancakes.

VARIATION: Skip the frosting and drizzle the pancakes with Keto Maple Syrup or top with whipped cream (here) and fresh berries.

PER SERVING (3 PANCAKES WITHOUT FROSTING): Calories: 334; Total fat: 30g; Total carbs: 7g; Fiber: 3.5g; Net carbs: 3.5g; Protein: 9g

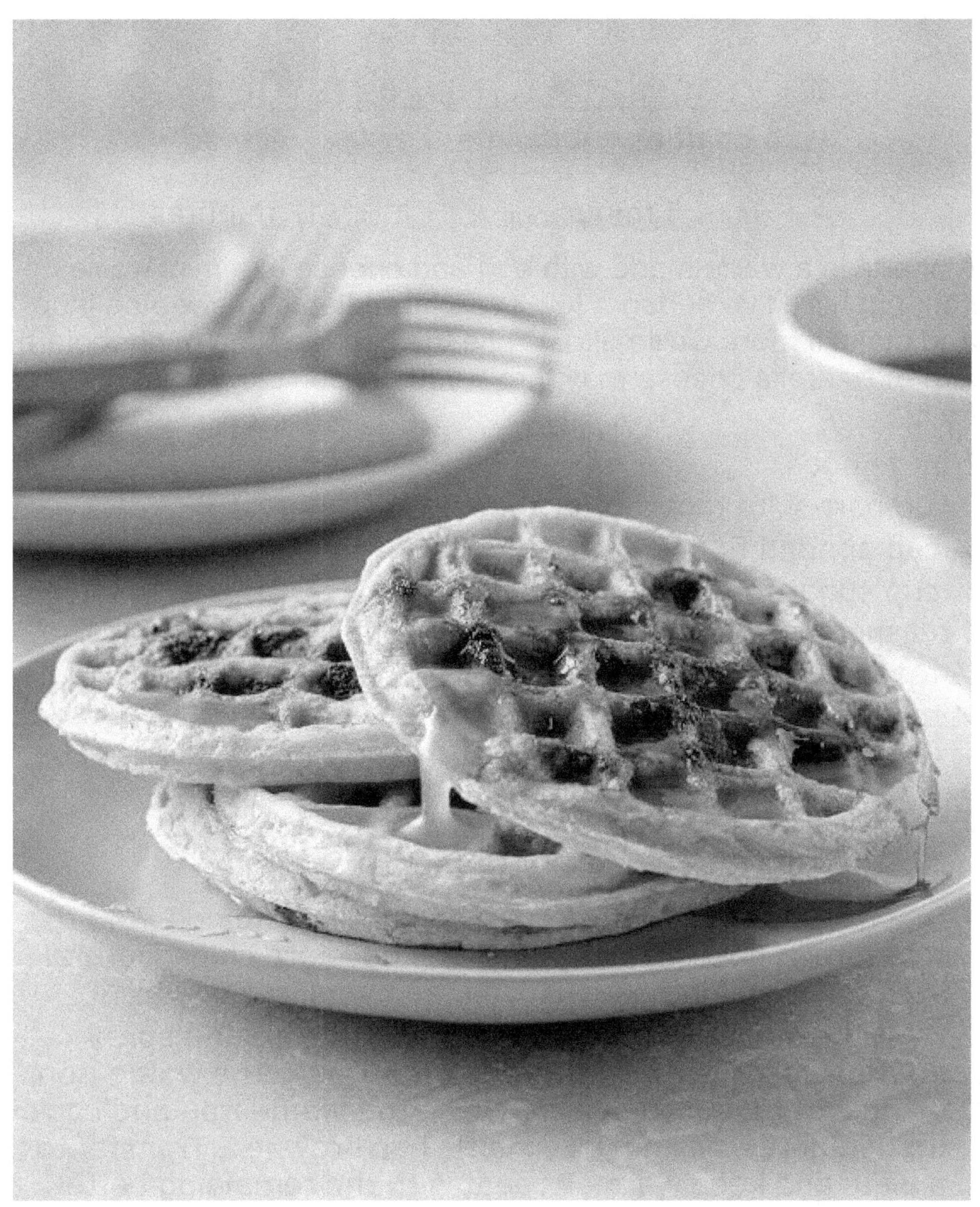

Chocolate Chip Chaffles

MAKES: **4 chaffles** | 30 Minutes or Less, Quick Prep, Vegetarian
PREP TIME: **5 minutes** | COOK TIME: **12 minutes**

A chaffle is a waffle made with egg and cheese in a mini waffle iron, but here I've added a few extra ingredients to sweeten it up and make it more waffle-like. While the combination of chocolate and mozzarella cheese may throw you off, don't knock it until you try it!

2 large eggs
1 cup part-skim mozzarella cheese
¼ cup almond flour
¼ cup sugar-free chocolate chips
1 teaspoon granulated natural sweetener
½ teaspoon baking powder
⅛ teaspoon salt
½ teaspoon pure vanilla extract
Olive oil cooking spray
¼ cup Keto Maple Syrup or store-bought, optional)

1. In a medium bowl, whisk the eggs until combined. Add the mozzarella cheese, almond flour, chocolate chips, natural sweetener, baking powder, salt, and vanilla. Stir well.
2. Heat the waffle iron until hot. Coat with cooking spray. Pour one-quarter of the chaffle batter onto the waffle iron, being careful not to overfill. Close the waffle iron and cook for 3 minutes, or until the chaffle has browned. Transfer to a plate and keep warm. Repeat with the remaining batter.

3. To serve, top each chaffle with 1 tablespoon of maple syrup (if using).

 For a different flavor profile, try sugar-free butterscotch, peanut butter or white chocolate chips instead of chocolate.

PER SERVING (2 CHAFFLES): Calories: 490; Total fat: 35g; Total carbs 24g; Fiber: 14g; Net carbs: 7g; Protein 25g

Raspberry Muffins

This is one of the first keto muffin recipes I created, and it's still a fan favorite. These muffins are best served cold and make an easy breakfast when you are on the go. They will last up to one week in the refrigerator and two months in the freezer.

1 cup almond flour

¼ cup coconut flour

⅔ cup granulated natural sweetener

2 teaspoons baking powder

¼ teaspoon salt

¼ cup unsalted butter, melted

¼ cup heavy (whipping) cream

¼ cup water

3 large eggs

1 teaspoon pure almond extract

1 cup fresh or frozen raspberries (if frozen, do not thaw
 before using)

1. Preheat the oven to 325°F. Line a 12-cup muffin pan with paper liners and set aside.

2. In a large bowl, mix the almond flour, coconut flour, natural sweetener, baking powder, and salt.

3. In a large microwave-safe bowl, heat the butter on High for 30 seconds or until just melted. To the melted butter, add the heavy cream, water, eggs, and almond extract. Whisk well.

4. Make a well in the center of the dry ingredients and pour the wet ingredients into the well. Using a wooden spoon, mix until the ingredients are thoroughly combined. Gently fold in the raspberries.

5. Fill each well of the prepared muffin pan with ¼ cup of the muffin batter. Bake for 30 minutes, or until the tops are lightly browned around the edges and a toothpick inserted into the center of a muffin comes out clean. Let cool completely.

6. Transfer the cooled muffins to an airtight container and refrigerate for up to 1 week and freeze for up to 2 to 3 months if needed.

PER SERVING (1 MUFFIN): Calories: 140; Total fat: 11g; Total carbs: 6.25g; Fiber: 2.5g; Net carbs: 4g; Protein: 4g

Layered Strawberry Chia Pudding

While chilling, chia seeds thicken the coconut milk to a pudding-like texture that's irresistibly good. You'll need to make the pudding at least a day before you intend to enjoy it, because it needs to chill for 12 hours before you layer it with the sauce.

FOR THE CHIA PUDDING

2 cups unsweetened almond milk

¼ cup chia seeds

1 tablespoon powdered natural sweetener

FOR THE STRAWBERRY SAUCE

3 cups fresh strawberries, hulled and diced

¼ cup granulated natural sweetener

½ (0.25-ounce) envelope unflavored gelatin

½ teaspoon pure vanilla extract

Pinch salt

TO MAKE THE CHIA PUDDING

1. In a large bowl, whisk together the almond milk and chia seeds. Stir in the natural sweetener. Cover and refrigerate for 12 hours.

TO MAKE THE STRAWBERRY SAUCE

2. In a large pot over medium-low heat, combine the strawberries, natural sweetener, and gelatin. Bring to a boil, and reduce the heat to low, cover with a lid, and simmer, stirring occasionally, for 15 minutes, until the natural sweetener has dissolved and the mixture has thickened.

3. Remove the strawberry sauce from the heat. Stir in the vanilla and salt. Set aside until cooled completely. Cover and refrigerate until ready to assemble the pudding.

TO SERVE

4. Divide the strawberry sauce evenly between 6 parfait dishes. Top with an even amount of the coconut chia mixture. Cover with plastic wrap and refrigerate until ready to serve.

PER SERVING: Calories: 51; Total fat: 3g; Total carbs: 4g; Fiber: 2.5g; Net carbs: 1.5g; Protein: 2g

Egg and Sausage Cauliflower Hash

SERVES: 4 | Dairy-Free, Quick Prep
PREP TIME: 10 minutes | COOK TIME: 30 minutes

My mom always would make eggs and hash for a weekend breakfast. Hash is normally made with leftover corned beef and potatoes, but to make this a quick and easy low-carb recipe, I substituted turkey sausage for the beef and cauliflower rice for the potatoes. I like to fry the eggs and serve them over the hash, but they can be scrambled and served alongside, if desired.

1 tablespoon extra-virgin olive oil, divided

½ cup diced onion

2 garlic cloves, minced

8 ounces turkey sausage or uncooked Homemade Breakfast Sausage

4 cups riced cauliflower

½ teaspoon salt

¼ teaspoon freshly ground black pepper

3 tablespoons coconut aminos

8 large eggs

1. In a large nonstick skillet over medium heat, heat 1 teaspoon of the olive oil. Add the onion and garlic, and cook, stirring often, for 3 minutes or until the onion becomes translucent.

2. Add the sausage and cook for 5 minutes or until the sausage is cooked through. Using a slotted spoon, transfer the sausage mixture to a plate.

3. Increase the heat to medium-high. Add the cauliflower to the pan, spreading it out evenly. Cook, without stirring, for

3 minutes or until the cauliflower is golden brown on the bottom. Stir in the salt, black pepper, and coconut aminos. Cover and cook for 3 minutes or until the cauliflower is tender and golden.

4. Return the sausage mixture to the skillet with the cauliflower, and stir to combine. Cook for 2 minutes, or until the sausage is heated through.

5. In another skillet over medium heat, heat 1 teaspoon of the olive oil. Crack 4 of the eggs into the pan and cook for 3 minutes, or until the yolks are still runny but the egg whites are set. Transfer the cooked eggs to a plate and keep warm. Repeat with the remaining olive oil and eggs.

6. To serve, divide the hash evenly between 4 plates. Top each with 2 eggs.

INGREDIENT TIP: Be sure to read the label when purchasing coconut aminos. Not all brands are lower in sugar content (and so will up the carbs in a recipe). Coconut Secret is my favorite keto-friendly brand.

PER SERVING: Calories: 341; Total fat: 23g; Total carbs: 9.5g; Fiber: 2.5g; Net carbs: 7g; Protein: 24g

Egg in a Hole Pepper Rings

SERVES: **2** | 5 Ingredients or Less, 30 Minutes or Less, One Pot, Quick Prep, Vegetarian
PREP TIME: **5 minutes** | COOK TIME: **5 minutes**

This is my colorful keto take on toad-in-a-hole, which is traditionally made with eggs and buttered bread. These are fun to serve for weekend brunch (the recipe can easily be doubled for a family of four) and are delicious with a drizzle of Chipotle Ranch Dressing.

Olive oil cooking spray

1 large red bell pepper, seeded, cored, and cut into 4 rings

4 large eggs

½ teaspoon salt

¼ teaspoon freshly ground black pepper

¼ cup shredded full-fat cheddar cheese

1 teaspoon chopped fresh basil leaves, for serving (optional)

1. Heat a large nonstick skillet over medium-high heat. Coat with cooking spray.

2. Place the bell pepper rings in the skillet and cook on one side for 2 minutes, or until the peppers start to brown. Flip each pepper ring over and reduce the heat to medium-low.

3. Carefully crack an egg into the center of each pepper ring. Season with salt and black pepper. Cover the pan with a tight-fitting lid and cook for 2 minutes or until the egg whites have set. Sprinkle each with the cheese, cover with the lid, and cook for 30 seconds or until the cheese has melted.

4. Sprinkle each egg pepper ring with chopped basil (if using) and serve.

INGREDIENT TIP: Use a variety of colored bell peppers for a rainbow breakfast. I like to use green, red, orange, and yellow. For a little added zing, omit the basil and make a quick mint dressing: whisk 1 teaspoon of finely chopped mint with 1 tablespoon lemon juice, season with salt and pepper to taste, and then drizzle it over the eggs prior to serving.

PER SERVING: Calories: 349; Total fat: 29g; Total carbs: 6g; Fiber: 1.5g; Net carbs: 4.5g; Protein: 16g

MusHroom CHeese Omelet

SERVES: **1** | 30 Minutes or Less, Quick Prep, Vegetarian
PREP TIME: **10 minutes** | COOK TIME: **10 minutes**

Eggs are my go-to in the morning. They are a good source of protein and contain no carbs. Omelets can be filled with more low-carb ingredients, adding both flavor and bulk. This is my favorite single-serving recipe for breakfast.

1 tablespoon unsalted butter

1 tablespoon diced yellow onion

1 cup sliced mushrooms

2 large eggs

¼ teaspoon garlic powder

¼ teaspoon salt

⅛ teaspoon freshly ground black pepper

¼ cup shredded full-fat cheddar cheese

1. In a large skillet over medium heat, heat the butter until melted and bubbling. Add the onion and cook for 2 minutes, until translucent. Add the mushrooms and cook for 5 minutes or until the mushrooms are lightly browned. Transfer the mixture to a bowl and set aside; reserve the skillet.

2. In a large bowl, whisk together the eggs, garlic powder, salt, and pepper. Pour the egg mixture into the reserved skillet. Cook over medium heat for 1 minute or until the eggs begin to set. Carefully flip the omelet over.

3. On one side of the egg, top with the mushroom mixture and cheese. Fold the omelet in half to cover the filling, and cook for 1 minute more or until the cheese begins to melt.

PER SERVING: Calories: 373; Total fat: 30g; Total carbs: 5g; Fiber: 1g; Net carbs: 4g; Protein: 21g

Eggs with Goat Cheese and Asparagus

SERVES: **2** | 5 Ingredients or Less, 30 Minutes or Less, One Pot, Quick Prep, Vegetarian

PREP TIME: **5 minutes** | COOK TIME: **6 minutes**

If you are not an asparagus fan, this dish may win you over! (Avoid any woody asparagus ends by bending each asparagus spear in your hand until it breaks. The asparagus spear will break where it is tender.) Garnish with parsley or herbs as desired.

1 tablespoon extra-virgin olive oil, divided

10 asparagus spears, trimmed

¼ teaspoon salt

⅛ teaspoon freshly ground black pepper

1 teaspoon fresh lemon juice

6 large eggs, whisked

2 ounces full-fat goat cheese, crumbled

1. In a large skillet over high heat, heat ½ tablespoon of the olive oil until hot. Add the asparagus spears and season with salt and pepper. Cook for 2 minutes, or just until tender-crisp, shaking the skillet periodically to cook the asparagus evenly on all sides. Transfer the cooked asparagus to a plate and set aside.

2. To the same skillet, add the remaining ½ tablespoon olive oil and heat until hot. Stir in the whisked eggs and cook until just set around the edges. Reduce the heat to medium-low and cook the eggs for 1 additional minute. Using a spatula, pull the eggs from the outer edges of the pan toward the center, about 1 inch, to allow the runny egg on top to flow to the bottom of the skillet. Continue cooking for 1 minute or until egg is almost set.

3. Sprinkle the goat cheese over the egg, and cook for 1 minute or until the egg is completely set. Divide the egg mixture between two plates and top with the cooked asparagus.

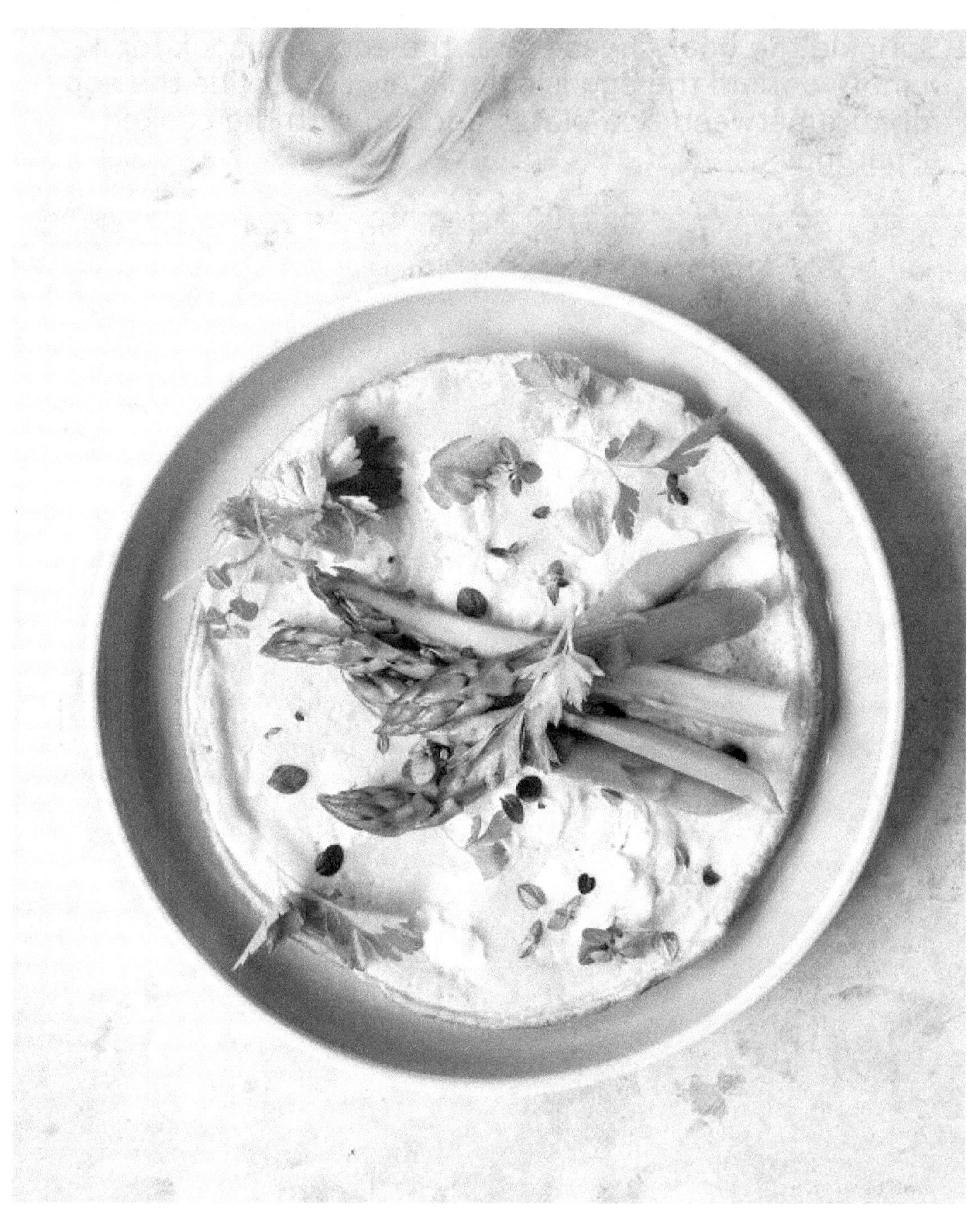

Loaded Breakfast Bowls

SERVES: **4** | 5 Ingredients or Less, 30 Minutes or Less, One Pot, Quick Prep

PREP TIME: **10 minutes** | COOK TIME: **20 minutes**

You'll be surprised at how well radishes sub in for potatoes in this tasty breakfast bowl. Cooking the radishes tames their spicy edge. You'll be hooked.

1 tablespoon extra-virgin olive oil, divided

2 cups fresh radishes, cubed

½ teaspoon garlic powder

½ teaspoon salt

¼ teaspoon freshly ground black pepper

8 ounces uncooked pork sausage, crumbled (or uncooked Homemade Breakfast Sausage)

6 large eggs, whisked

½ cup shredded full-fat cheddar cheese

1. In a large skillet over medium heat, heat ½ tablespoon of the olive oil until it shimmers. Add the radishes and season with the garlic powder, salt, and pepper. Cook for 7 minutes, stirring occasionally, until the radishes are easily pierced with a fork. Transfer the cooked radishes to a medium bowl and set aside.

2. To the same skillet, add the sausage and cook, stirring often, for 7 minutes or until browned and cooked through. Transfer to the bowl of cooked radishes. Set aside.

3. Wipe the skillet clean and add the remaining olive oil. Heat over medium heat until it shimmers. Add the whisked eggs and cook for 1 minute or until the eggs begin to set.

4. Reduce the heat to medium-low. Using a rubber spatula, pull the eggs across the bottom of the pan to form large, soft curds. Continue to cook for 3 minutes, folding and stirring the eggs until the eggs are cooked to your liking.

5. Return the sausage and radish mixture to the skillet and stir to combine. Remove the pan from the heat. Sprinkle the cheese over the eggs. Cover the pan with a lid and set aside for 1 minute, until the cheese has melted. Serve.

PER SERVING: Calories: 350; Total fat: 26g; Total carbs: 7g; Fiber: 1.5g; Net carbs: 5.5g; Protein: 22g

Homemade Breakfast Sausage

MAKES: **10 sausage patties** | 5 Ingredients or Less, 30 Minutes or Less, Dairy-Free, Quick Prep
PREP TIME: **10 minutes** | COOK TIME: **6 minutes**

You can make these flavorful breakfast sausages ahead and store them in the freezer. Just layer uncooked sausage patties between sheets of parchment paper and place in an airtight container. They will keep, frozen, for up to 3 months. To cook, add a frozen patty to a pan and cook over medium-low heat for 10 minutes, turning often, until browned and cooked through.

12 ounces ground turkey

6 ounces ground pork

1 tablespoon chopped fresh sage leaves

2 teaspoons chopped fresh thyme leaves

1 teaspoon fennel seeds, crushed

½ teaspoon red pepper flakes (optional)

½ teaspoon salt

¼ teaspoon freshly ground black pepper

1. In a large bowl, combine the turkey, pork, sage, thyme, crushed fennel seeds, red pepper flakes (if using), salt, and pepper. Mix until well combined.

2. Scoop ¼ cup of the meat mixture into your hands and form a patty about ½ inch thick. Repeat with the remaining mixture. You should end up with 10 equal-size patties.

3. Heat a large skillet over medium-high heat. Place the sausage patties in the hot skillet (you may need to cook them in batches so as not to crowd the pan) and cook for 3 minutes, until the bottoms are browned. Flip each patty

over and cook for another 3 minutes or until the sausage is browned and cooked through to an internal temperature of 145°F.

COOKING TIP: An air fryer is an excellent way to cook these sausage patties with no grease splatter! Just place the patties in the air fryer and cook at 375°F for 15 minutes or until the internal temperature of the patties is at 145°F.

PER SERVING (2 PATTIES): Calories: 142; Total fat: 6.5g; Total carbs: 0g; Fiber: 0g; Net carbs: 0g; Protein: 21g

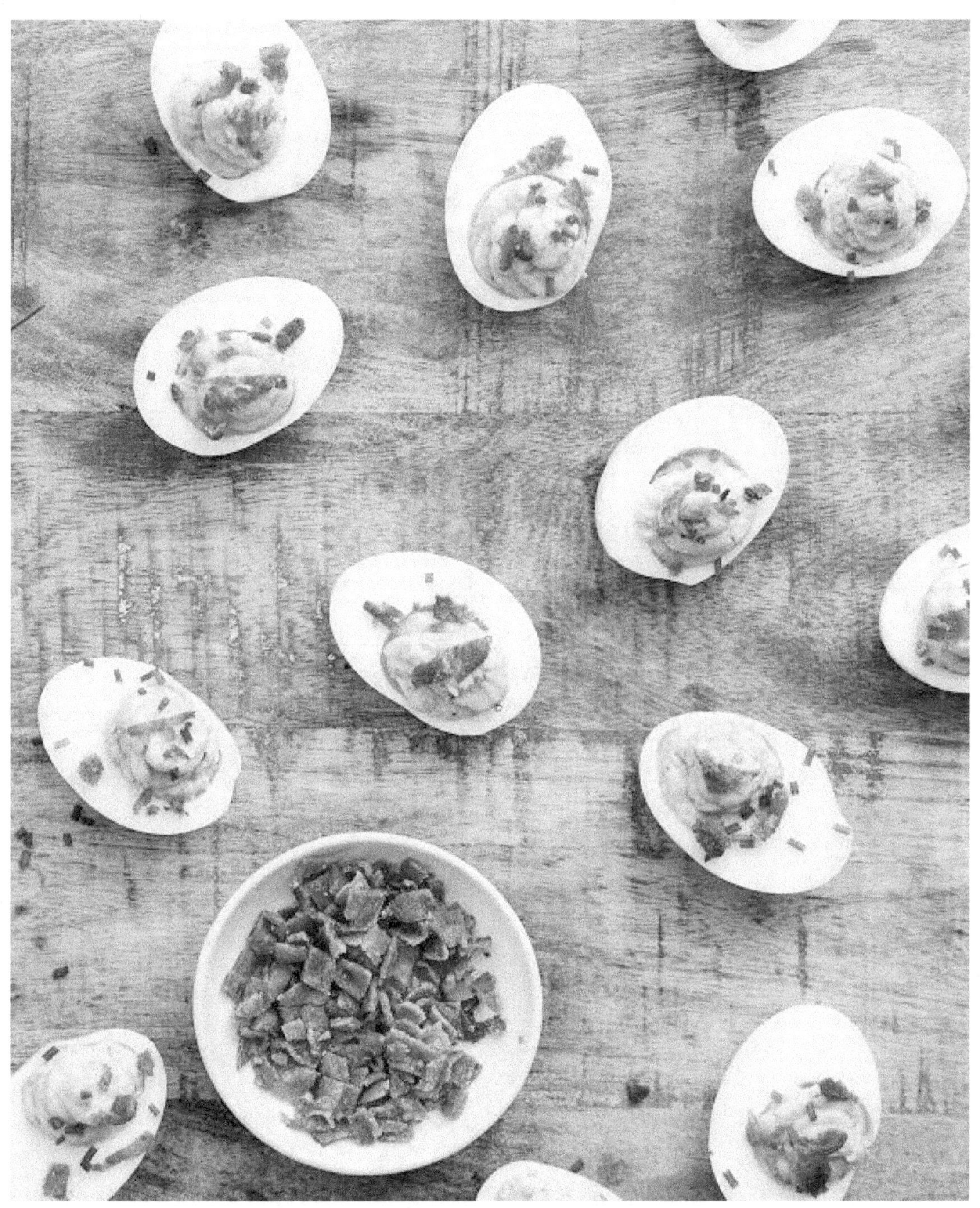
Loaded Deviled Eggs

4

Snacks and Sides

Buffalo Chicken Dip
Swiss Onion Dip
Zucchini Fries
Creamy Coleslaw
Keto Hummus
Glazed Mushrooms
Onion Rings
Cauliflower Fried Rice
Loaded Deviled Eggs
Pulled Pork–Stuffed Mushrooms

Buffalo Chicken Dip

MAKES: **4 cups** | Quick Prep
PREP TIME: **10 minutes** | COOK TIME: **30 minutes**

This recipe makes a great game-day appetizer. You can even make it with leftover cooked chicken or canned chicken. For the hot sauce, I like to use Frank's Red Hot, but feel free to use your favorite brand of wing sauce so long as it is keto-friendly. I like to serve this dip with carrot, celery, cucumber, and bell pepper strips.

Olive oil cooking spray

1 package (8 ounces) cream cheese, softened

¼ cup keto-friendly ranch dressing

½ cup hot sauce

1 cup shredded full-fat cheddar cheese

3 scallions, sliced, white and green parts separated

2 cups cooked chicken

½ cup full-fat crumbly blue cheese

1. Preheat the oven to 350°F. Coat an 8-by-8-inch baking dish with the cooking spray and set aside.
2. In a medium-sized mixing bowl, using an electric mixer, combine the cream cheese and ranch dressing until smooth.
3. Add the hot sauce, cheddar cheese, and white part of the scallion. Mix until smooth. Using a wooden spoon, fold in the cooked chicken until coated with the cheese mixture.
4. Transfer the chicken mixture to the prepared baking dish, spreading evenly. Sprinkle the crumbly blue cheese evenly over the top. Bake for 30 minutes or until bubbling.

5. Remove the pan from the oven. Sprinkle the dip with the
   green parts of the scallions. Serve hot.

COOKING TIP: You can cook this in a slow cooker. Simply
combine the ingredients as in steps 2 and 3, then transfer the
mixture to the bowl of a slow cooker. Cover with the lid and
cook on high for 1½ hours or until hot all the way through.
Sprinkle with the scallions. Serve hot.

PER SERVING (½ CUP): Calories: 288; Total fat: 24g; Total carbs:
3g; Fiber: 0g; Net carbs: 3g; Protein: 15g

Swiss Onion Dip

MAKES: **4 cups** | Quick Prep, Vegetarian
PREP TIME: **10 minutes** | COOK TIME: **30 minutes**

Serve this dip at tailgate parties or as a holiday appetizer. It's delicious served warm with halved mini bell peppers for scooping. Although onion intake should be limited on keto, this recipe only yields a few carbs per serving. I like to use Vidalia onions for this recipe, which are milder, but white onions can be used as well.

2 cups chopped Vidalia onion

2 cups shredded full-fat Swiss cheese

4 ounces full-fat cream cheese, softened

½ cup keto-friendly mayonnaise or Avocado Oil Mayonnaise

2 tablespoons prepared horseradish (optional)

1½ teaspoons hot sauce (optional)

1 teaspoon smoked paprika

1. Preheat the oven to 375°F. Set aside a deep-dish pie plate or 8-by-8-inch baking dish.

2. In a large mixing bowl, using an electric mixer, combine the onion, Swiss cheese, cream cheese, mayonnaise, horseradish (if using), and hot sauce (if using).

3. Transfer the mixture to the pie plate or baking dish. Sprinkle with the paprika and bake for 30 minutes or until the dip is bubbling around the edges and hot in the center.

COOKING TIP: If you prefer, you can cook this in a slow cooker. In step 3, transfer the mixture to the slow cooker. Sprinkle with the paprika. Cover with the lid and cook on high for 1½ hours or until the dip is hot all the way through.

PER SERVING (¼ CUP): Calories: 134; Total fat: 12g; Total carbs: 2.5g; Fiber: 0.5g; Net carbs: 2g; Protein: 4g

ZuccHini Fries

SERVES: **4** | 5 Ingredients or Less, Dairy-Free, Vegetarian
PREP TIME: **20 minutes** | COOK TIME: **15 minutes**

Zucchini fries may seem like a lot of work, but they are worth it. My version is baked as a healthier option, but if you like a crispier fry, feel free to deep-fry the zucchini in extra-virgin olive oil instead. Try them with a side of Fry Dipping Sauce.

Olive oil cooking spray, divided

1 large egg, beaten

1 tablespoon water

⅔ cup almond meal

½ teaspoon salt

½ teaspoon garlic powder

2 small zucchinis, cut into strips or rounds

1. Preheat the oven to 350°F. Line a baking pan with parchment paper and spray with the cooking spray. Set aside.

2. In a medium bowl, whisk together the egg and water.

3. In another medium bowl, stir together the almond meal, salt, and garlic powder.

4. Dip the zucchini first in the egg batter, and then in the almond meal mixture, being sure to coat each piece completely. Place the coated fries on the prepared baking sheet. Repeat with the remaining ingredients. Lightly spray the top of the fries with cooking spray.

5. Bake for 7 minutes, or until the zucchini fries begin to brown. Remove the pan from the oven and, using a spatula, turn the fries over. Return the pan to the oven and bake for

another 7 minutes, until the zucchini fries are browned and cooked through. Remove the pan from the oven and serve fries while still hot.

INGREDIENT TIP: Almond meal is similar to almond flour but is a little coarser. Feel free to use almond flour or pecan meal if that is what you have.

PER SERVING: Calories: 156; Total fat: 14g; Total carbs: 3.5g; Fiber: 2g; Net carbs: 1.5g; Protein: 4g

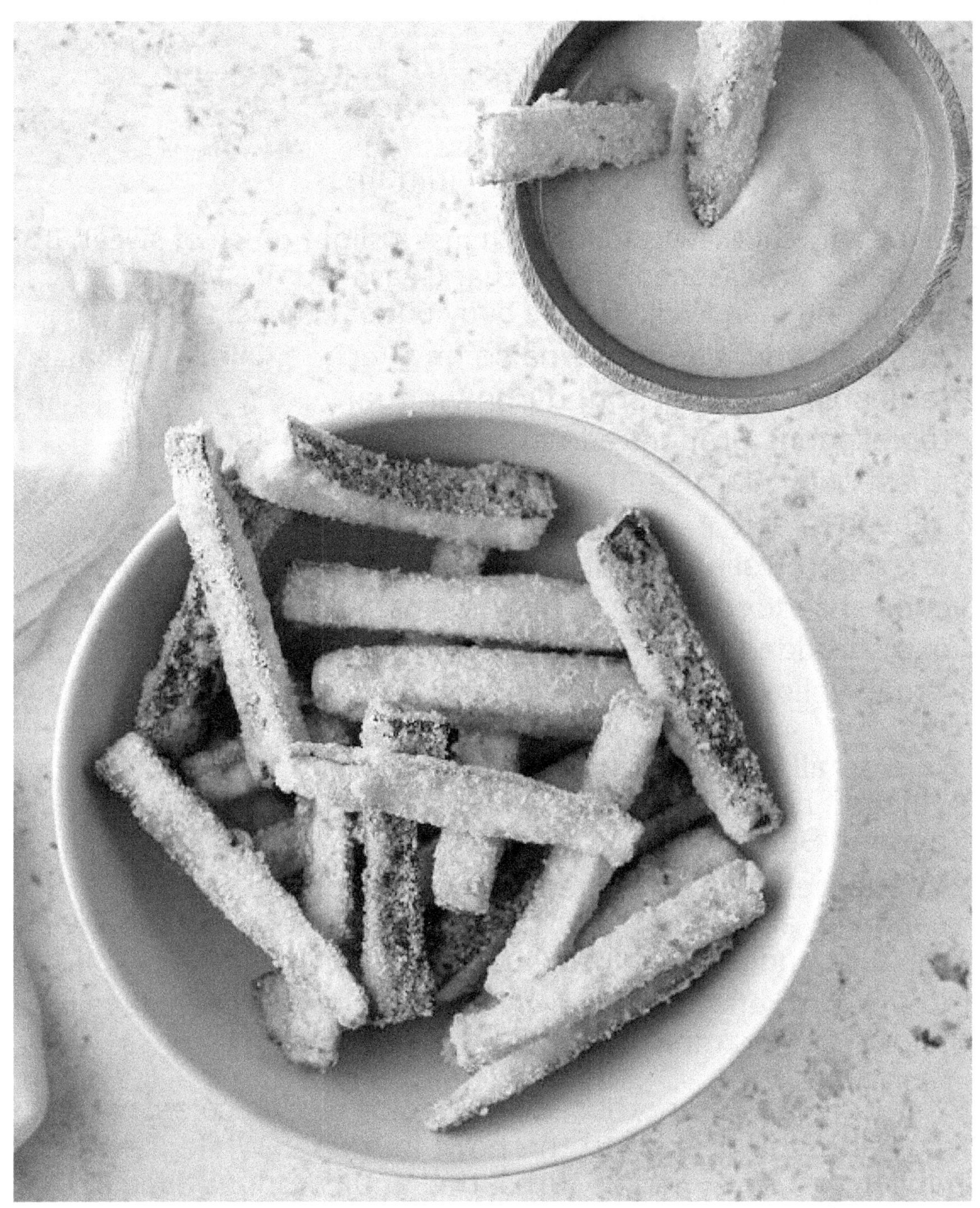

Creamy Coleslaw

This creamy coleslaw is tangy with just a slight touch of sweet. Be sure to use unseasoned rice vinegar (seasoned rice vinegar contains sugar and will kick the body out of ketosis, see here).

¾ cup keto-friendly mayonnaise or Avocado Oil Mayonnaise

2 tablespoons unseasoned rice vinegar

2 tablespoons granulated natural sweetener (optional)

½ teaspoon celery seed

½ teaspoon salt

¼ teaspoon freshly ground black pepper

3 cups shredded green cabbage

1 cup shredded purple cabbage

¼ small yellow onion, finely diced

1. In a small bowl, whisk together the mayonnaise, rice vinegar, natural sweetener (if using), celery seed, salt, and pepper. Set aside.

2. In a large bowl, combine the green cabbage, purple cabbage, and onion. Pour the dressing over the cabbage mixture and toss until well coated.

3. Cover and refrigerate the coleslaw for up to three days to let the flavors meld.

VARIATION: To add another level of color to this coleslaw, add ¼ cup shredded carrot to the bowl in step 2. While it's true that carrots are higher in carbs, the small amount used in this recipe will not drastically change the carb count.

PER SERVING (½ CUP): Calories: 158; Total fat: 16g; Total carbs: 3g; Fiber: 1g; Net carbs: 2g; Protein: 0.5g

Keto Hummus

MAKES: **4 cups** | Dairy-Free, Quick Prep, Vegetarian, Worth the Wait

PREP TIME: **10 minutes** | COOK TIME: **35 minutes**

Roasting the cauliflower and garlic adds a delicious flavor profile to this recipe. It is more time-consuming to prepare, but absolutely worth the wait. If you are in a hurry, save on prep time by purchasing a 1-pound bag of cauliflower florets instead of breaking down the cauliflower.

½ cup extra-virgin olive oil, divided

1 large head cauliflower, cut into florets

½ cup tahini

3 garlic cloves, chopped

1 teaspoon ground cumin

½ teaspoon freshly ground black pepper

½ teaspoon salt

¼ teaspoon cayenne pepper (optional)

1. Preheat the oven to 400°F. Set aside a large baking sheet.

2. In a large bowl, add ¼ cup of the olive oil. Add the cauliflower florets and toss until well coated. Spread the mixture evenly over the baking sheet. Roast for 35 minutes or until the cauliflower is browned and can be easily pierced with a fork.

3. Transfer the roasted cauliflower to the bowl of a food processor. Add the remaining olive oil, tahini, garlic, cumin, pepper, salt, and cayenne pepper (if using). Cover with the lid and process on high until smooth and creamy, scraping

down the sides of the bowl as needed. Transfer the mixture to a bowl and let cool (or refrigerate) before serving.

TIME-SAVING TIP: To save time in step 3, steam the cauliflower instead of roasting it. Place the cauliflower in a steamer on the stove or in the microwave and cook until fork tender. Proceed to step 4.

PER SERVING (¼ CUP): Calories: 123; Total fat: 11g; Total carbs: 4g; Fiber: 1.5g; Net carbs: 3g; Protein: 2g

Glazed Mushrooms

SERVES: **4** | 5 Ingredients or Less, One Pot, Quick Prep, Vegetarian
PREP TIME: **10 minutes** | COOK TIME: **10 minutes**

Sautéed mushrooms are delicious, but these glazed mushrooms bring the fungi experience to a whole new level! Red pepper flakes add a small amount of heat while coconut aminos cook down to a sweet glaze. It's the best kind of sweet heat. If you are a little timid of the heat, reduce the amount of red pepper flakes to ¼ teaspoon or omit altogether.

2 tablespoons salted butter

16 ounces button mushrooms, quartered

2 tablespoons coconut aminos

½ teaspoon red pepper flakes (optional)

1. In a large skillet over medium-high heat, melt the butter and heat until bubbling.
2. Add the mushrooms and cook, stirring occasionally, for 5 minutes, until the mushrooms have softened and released their liquid.
3. Stir in the coconut aminos and red pepper flakes (if using). Continue to cook the mushrooms for 4 minutes or until any liquid in the pan has evaporated. Serve warm.

VARIATION: In step 3, omit the coconut aminos and instead add ½ teaspoon garlic powder. Add ¼ cup dry red wine and cook for 4 minutes, scraping up any brown bits on the bottom of the pan, until any liquid has been cooked off.

PER SERVING: Calories: 86; Total fat: 6g; Total carbs: 5g; Fiber: 1g; Net carbs: 4g; Protein: 3g

Onion Rings

Onions are higher in carbs so should be limited on keto, but who can resist a good onion ring dipped in Fry Dipping Sauce? Vidalia onions are milder but do have a higher sugar content. Feel free to substitute yellow onions.

Olive oil cooking spray, divided

1 cup almond flour

1 cup grated Parmesan cheese

1 teaspoon smoked paprika

½ teaspoon salt

¼ teaspoon freshly ground black pepper

2 eggs

1 tablespoon water

1 large Vidalia onion, cut into rings

1. Preheat the oven to 400°F. Line a baking sheet with parchment paper and spray with cooking spray. Set aside.
2. In a medium bowl, combine the almond flour, Parmesan, paprika, salt, and pepper. In a small bowl, whisk together the eggs and water.
3. Dip each onion ring first into the egg mixture, and then into the flour mixture, being sure to coat each piece completely. Place the coated rings on the prepared baking sheet. Lightly spray the tops of the onion rings with cooking spray.

4. Bake for 10 minutes, or until the onion rings begin to brown on the bottoms. Remove the pan from the oven and, using a spatula, turn each onion ring over. Lightly spray the rings with more cooking spray. Bake for another 10 minutes, until the onion rings have browned. Remove the pan from the oven and serve the onion rings while still hot.

FLAVOR BOOST: **To add a Buffalo-style flavor to the onion rings, substitute an equal amount of hot sauce for the water in the egg mixture.**

PER SERVING: Calories: 193; Total fat: 15g; Total carbs: 7.5g; Fiber: 2g; Net carbs: 5.5g; Protein: 7g

Cauliflower Fried Rice

SERVES: **4** | 5 Ingredients or Less, 30 Minutes or Less, Dairy-Free, One Pot, Quick Prep, Vegetarian
PREP TIME: **10 minutes** | COOK TIME: **15 minutes**

This is a great side dish that goes with just about any protein you plan to serve. Use your food processor to quickly and easily rice florets of cauliflower. To save on prep time, you can substitute 4 cups of pre-riced cauliflower. If desired, you can substitute an equal amount of soy sauce for the coconut aminos.

2 tablespoons extra-virgin olive oil

½ small onion, diced

2 garlic cloves, minced

1 head cauliflower, riced

1 tablespoon coconut aminos

1 teaspoon salt

½ teaspoon freshly ground black pepper

1. In a large skillet over medium-high heat, heat the olive oil until it shimmers. Add the onion and garlic, and cook, stirring occasionally, for 3 minutes or until the onion begins to turn translucent.

2. Add the cauliflower to the onions and stir until well combined. Cover the pan with a lid and cook for 5 minutes without stirring.

3. Remove the lid and stir. Continue to cook, uncovered, for 5 minutes or until the cauliflower is tender.

4. Remove the pan from the heat. Stir in the coconut aminos, and season with salt and pepper. Serve.

VARIATION: Make a Spanish-style "rice" by adding ½ teaspoon each of chili powder, cumin powder, and garlic powder to the pan along with 2 tablespoons of tomato paste in step 1. In step 4, omit the coconut aminos.

PER SERVING (¾ CUP): Calories: 111; Total fat: 7g; Total carbs: 9g; Fiber: 3g; Net carbs: 6g; Protein: 3g

Loaded Deviled Eggs

Deviled eggs are a great way to add protein and fat to your diet. I like to hard-boil eggs ahead of time and keep them chilled in the refrigerator for a quick assembly. To get perfectly hard-boiled eggs, place the eggs in a saucepan and cover with an inch of cold water. Bring the water to a boil, and then immediately turn off the heat. Cover the pan with a lid and set aside for 15 minutes. Drain the water from the pan, let the eggs cool, and peel.

12 large hard-boiled eggs, shelled, halved, and yolks reserved

1 cup keto-friendly mayonnaise or Avocado Oil Mayonnaise

1 tablespoon spicy brown mustard

2 garlic cloves, minced

½ teaspoon cayenne pepper

1 teaspoon smoked paprika

6 slices cooked sugar-free uncured bacon, crumbled (optional)

1. Place the egg yolks in a small bowl and mash with a fork. Add the mayonnaise, mustard, garlic, and cayenne pepper. Stir until combined.

2. Using a teaspoon, fill each egg half with the yolk mixture. Sprinkle each egg half with paprika and cooked bacon (if using). Serve immediately or cover and refrigerate until using. Deviled eggs will keep in the refrigerator for up to 2 days.

PER SERVING (2 EGG HALVES): Calories: 201; Total fat: 19g; Total carbs: 1g; Fiber: 0g; Net carbs: 1g; Protein: 6.5g

Pulled Pork–Stuffed Mushrooms

SERVES: **4** | 30 Minutes or Less, Quick Prep
PREP TIME: **10 minutes** | COOK TIME: **20 minutes**

Turn to this winning recipe when you have leftover Pulled Pork. The mushroom cap acts as a delicious vessel. You can also top these cooked mushrooms with Creamy Coleslaw for a delicious open-face-style sandwich.

1 cup Pulled Pork

4 ounces full-fat cream cheese, softened

1 jalapeño pepper, diced

2 tablespoons diced yellow onion

½ cup sugar-free barbecue sauce

4 large portobello mushroom caps, stems removed, and
 gills scraped out

¼ cup shredded full-fat cheddar cheese

1 cup Creamy Coleslaw, optional)

1. Preheat the oven to 375°F. Line a baking sheet with parchment paper and set aside.

2. Place the pulled pork in a microwave-safe dish and heat on high for 30-second bursts until the pork is warmed through, stirring between cook times.

3. Add the cream cheese, jalapeño, onion, and barbecue sauce. Stir until well combined.

4. Divide the pulled pork mixture into four even portions. Fill each mushroom cap with one portion of the pulled pork filling and place on the prepared baking sheet. Sprinkle each stuffed mushroom with 1 tablespoon shredded cheese.

5. Bake for 20 minutes, just until the cheese melts and the filling is warmed through. Remove the pan from the oven. To serve, top each mushroom with ¼ cup of coleslaw (if using).

INGREDIENT TIP: My preferred sugar-free barbecue sauce is G. Hughes Carolina Style. For a different flavor profile, you can substitute with Chipotle Ranch Dressing.

PER SERVING (1 MUSHROOM): Calories: 217; Total fat: 15g; Total carbs: 9.5g; Fiber: 2g; Net carbs: 7.5g; Protein: 11g

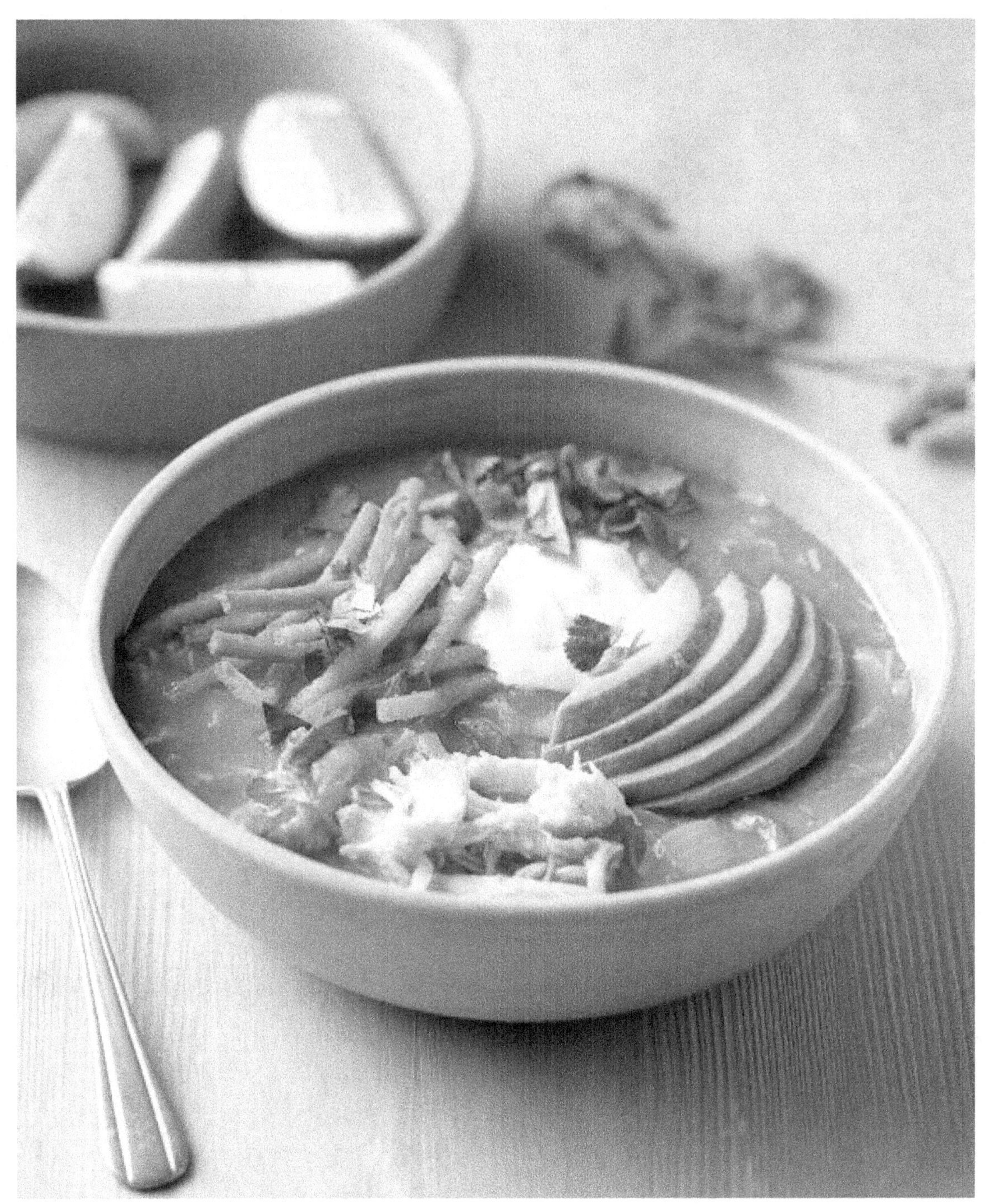

Chicken Tortilla Soup

5

<u>Soups and Salads</u>

<u>Chicken Tortilla Soup</u>
<u>Creamy Chicken Mushroom Soup</u>
<u>Butternut Squash Soup</u>
<u>Turkey Squash Soup</u>
<u>Keto-Style Broccoli Dal Soup</u>
<u>Italian Wedding Soup</u>
<u>Egg and Olive Salad</u>
<u>Garlic Shrimp, Asparagus, and Cilantro Salad</u>
<u>Keto Cobb Salad</u>
<u>Roasted Cauliflower Salad</u>
<u>Sweet and Spicy Broccoli Salad</u>
<u>Steak Salad</u>

Chicken Tortilla Soup

SERVES: 4 | Dairy-Free, Worth the Wait
PREP TIME: 30 minutes | COOK TIME: 5 hours, plus 10 minutes to cool

This is one of my favorite slow cooker recipes. Top this soup with lime, fresh cilantro, full-fat sour cream, and avocado, if desired.

1 (14.5-ounce) can diced tomatoes, with juice
½ (4½-ounce) can diced green chilies, with juice
¼ cup diced yellow onion
½ cup celery, chopped
2 garlic cloves, minced
1 pound boneless, skinless chicken breasts
1½ teaspoons chili powder
1 teaspoon ground cumin
1 teaspoon dried oregano
¾ teaspoon salt
½ teaspoon freshly ground black pepper
4 cups reduced-sodium chicken broth
½ cup extra-virgin olive oil
2 Cauliflower Tortillas, cut into strips

1. Combine the tomatoes, green chilies, onion, celery, and garlic in the slow cooker.

2. Arrange the chicken breasts in a single layer on top of the vegetables, and sprinkle with the chili powder, cumin, oregano, salt, and pepper. Pour in the chicken broth. Cover with the lid and cook on high for 5 hours. Transfer the chicken to a bowl and let cool for 10 minutes.

3. Transfer half of the soup to a blender. Blend until smooth. Return the blended soup to the crock pot, keeping it on warm.

4. Using two forks, shred the chicken and return to the slow cooker.

5. In a frying pan over medium-high heat, heat the olive oil until it shimmers. Add the tortilla strips and fry for 2 minutes, stirring often, until browned and crispy. Using a slotted spoon, transfer the strips to a paper towel to drain.

6. Serve the soup topped with crispy tortilla strips.

VARIATION: For a spicier soup, add 1 jalapeno pepper, seeded and cut into rings, in step 1.

PER SERVING (1¼ CUPS): Calories: 391; Total fat: 23g; Total carbs: 14g; Fiber: 4g; Net carbs: 10g; Protein: 32g

Creamy Chicken Mushroom Soup

SERVES: 6 | 30 Minutes or Less, One Pot, Quick Prep
PREP TIME: 10 minutes | COOK TIME: 15 minutes

Tangy cream cheese adds a richness to this soup, taking the place of flour and heavy cream. For best results, be sure to soften the cream cheese before adding it to the soup (heat it in the microwave for 15 seconds, if necessary).

4 tablespoons unsalted butter, divided

1 pound chicken breast tenders

1 teaspoon salt

½ teaspoon freshly ground black pepper

10 fresh sage leaves, minced

½ cup diced yellow onion

3 garlic cloves, minced

16 ounces fresh button mushrooms, sliced

8 ounces cream cheese, softened

4 cups reduced-sodium chicken broth

1. In a large pot over medium heat, heat 2 tablespoons of the butter until bubbling. Add the chicken tenders, salt, and pepper, and cook for 5 minutes on each side or until the tenders are browned and cooked through. Transfer the chicken to a plate and set aside.

2. Add the remaining 2 tablespoons of butter to the pot, and heat until bubbling. Add the sage and cook for 1 minute or until it begins to crisp.

3. Add the onion, garlic, and mushrooms. Cook, stirring for 5 minutes or until the mushrooms have softened and released their liquid.

4. Meanwhile, cut the chicken tenders into bite-size pieces.

5. Add the cream cheese to the mushroom mixture. Simmer for 2 minutes, stirring constantly, until the cream cheese is well incorporated into the mushroom mixture.

6. Return the cooked chicken to the soup. Stir in the chicken broth. Bring the soup to a boil, and then reduce heat and simmer for 2 minutes.

PER SERVING (1½ CUPS): Calories: 327; Total fat: 23g; Total carbs: 7g; Fiber: 1g; Net carbs: 6g; Protein: 23g

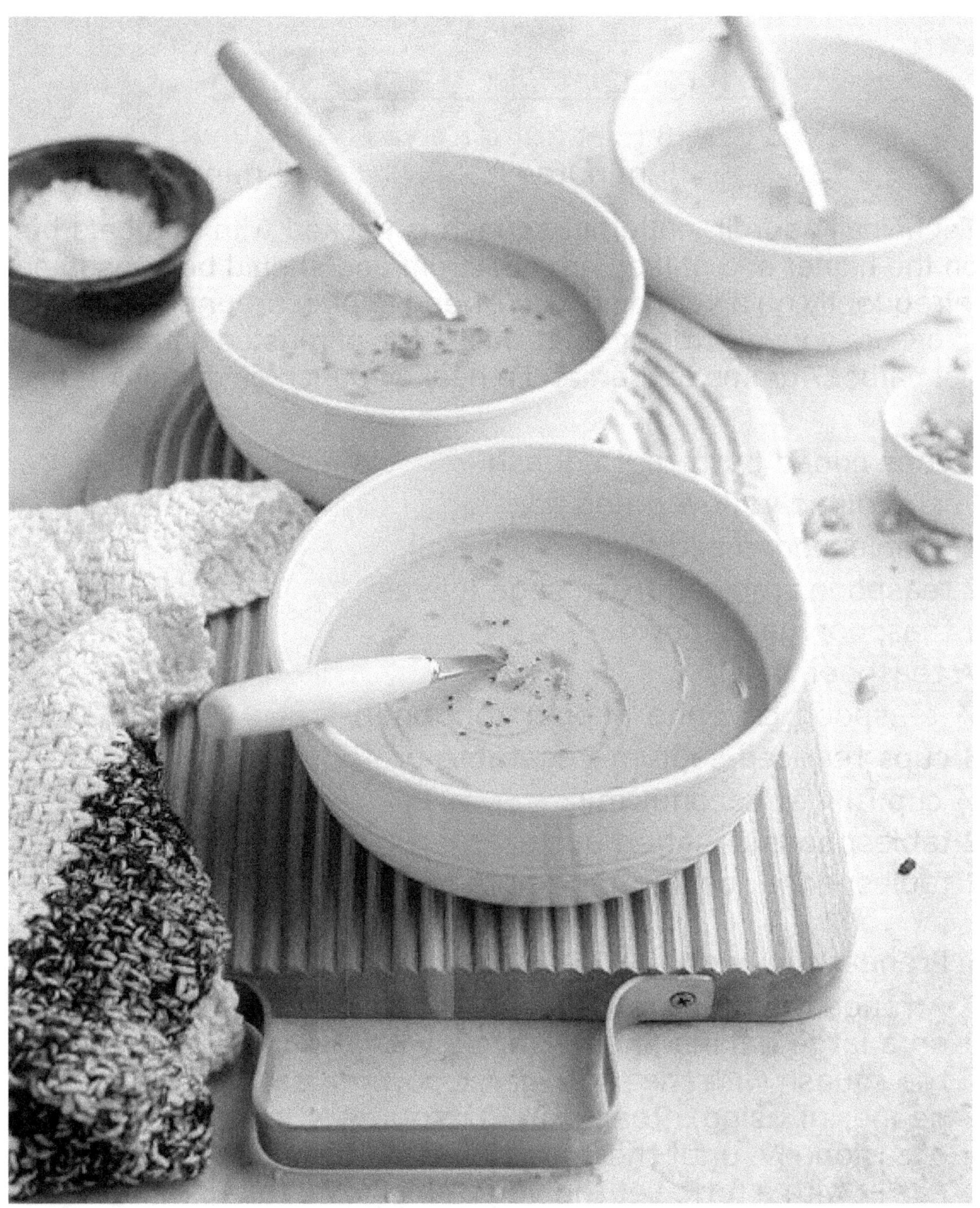

Butternut Squash Soup

SERVES: **8** | Vegetarian, Worth the Wait
PREP TIME: **15 minutes** | COOK TIME: **40 minutes**

Technically a fruit, butternut squash is packed with nutrients but on the higher end of the carb spectrum and should be consumed infrequently on a keto diet. You'll need to plan around this recipe to ensure your macros are met. Just 1 cup of roasted squash has 9 net carbs, 7 grams of fiber, and a healthy punch of vitamins A and C.

4 cups cubed butternut squash

½ cup diced yellow onion

1½ tablespoons extra-virgin olive oil

2 teaspoons minced fresh sage leaves

1 teaspoon garlic powder

½ teaspoon salt

¼ teaspoon cayenne pepper (optional)

3 cups reduced-sodium vegetable broth

½ cup full-fat coconut milk

2 tablespoons unsalted butter

2 tablespoons toasted pine nuts (optional)

1. Preheat the oven to 425°F.

2. Arrange the butternut squash and onion in a single layer on a large baking sheet. Drizzle with the olive oil. Season the squash with the sage, garlic powder, salt, and cayenne pepper (if using). Roast for 30 minutes, stirring occasionally, until the squash has softened and pierces easily with a fork. Let the vegetables cool for 15 minutes.

3. Transfer the roasted squash and onions to a blender. Add
   the vegetable broth and coconut milk. Cover with the lid
   and blend on high for 3 minutes or until the mixture is
   smooth. Transfer the puréed squash mixture to a large pot
   and keep warm.

4. In a small skillet over medium-high, heat the butter until
   bubbly. Serve each portion of soup drizzled with ½
   tablespoon of the butter and sprinkled with ½ tablespoon
   of the toasted pine nuts (if using).

COOKING TIP: Instead of roasting the squash, you can boil it
until tender. Then add the boiled squash with the seasonings
to the blender and proceed as instructed in step 4.

PER SERVING (1 CUP): Calories: 119; Total fat: 8.5g; Total carbs:
11g; Fiber: 2g; Net carbs: 9g; Protein: 1g

Turkey Squash Soup

SERVES: 6 | Dairy-Free, One Pot

PREP TIME: 15 minutes | COOK TIME: 25 minutes

This dish combines some of my favorite keto-friendly ingredients in soup form. Cooking the diced radishes with the garlic and onion transforms them into potato-like morsels. If you prefer a more peppery flavor, substitute an equal amount of baby arugula for the spinach.

1 tablespoon extra-virgin olive oil

8 ounces radishes, diced

½ cup diced yellow onion

2 garlic cloves, minced

1 pound ground turkey

1 teaspoon salt

½ teaspoon freshly ground black pepper

1 medium zucchini, chopped

1 carrot, shredded

8 cups reduced-sodium chicken broth

3 cups packed baby spinach

1. In a large pot over medium-high heat, heat the olive oil until it shimmers. Add the radishes, onion, and garlic, and sauté for 4 minutes, until the radishes begin to soften.

2. Crumble the ground turkey into the radish mixture. Cook, using a wooden spoon to break up the turkey, for 7 minutes, just until the turkey begins to brown.

3. Season the turkey with the salt and pepper, and cook for another 5 minutes, until the turkey is cooked through.

4. Stir in the zucchini, carrot, and chicken broth, and bring the mixture to a boil. Reduce the heat to medium-low and simmer for 10 minutes.

5. Stir in the spinach, and cook for 2 minutes, just until the spinach has wilted.

FLAVOR BOOST: You can also roast the radishes for a slightly different flavor: Preheat the oven to 400°F. Cut the radishes into quarters and toss with the onion, garlic, and olive oil on a baking sheet. Roast for 20 minutes. Add them to the turkey in step 3, with the salt and pepper.

PER SERVING (2 CUPS): Calories: 175; Total fat: 8g; Total carbs: 7g; Fiber: 1.5g; Net carbs: 5.5g; Protein: 19g

Keto-Style Broccoli Dal Soup

SERVES: **6** | 30 Minutes or Less, Dairy-Free, One Pot,
Vegetarian
PREP TIME: **15 minutes** | COOK TIME: **15 minutes**

Broccoli dal is an Indian dish traditionally made with lentils, but this version calls for riced cauliflower to reduce the carbs. Be careful and watch the mustard seeds when frying: they will quickly start popping in the pan.

2 tablespoons extra-virgin olive oil

2 teaspoons yellow mustard seeds

2 teaspoons cumin seeds

½ cup chopped yellow onion

4 cups riced cauliflower

1½ teaspoons yellow curry powder

1 teaspoon ground turmeric

1 teaspoon ground cumin

1 teaspoon salt

4 cups coarsely chopped broccoli

5 cups reduced-sodium vegetable broth

2 cups full-fat coconut milk

1. In a large soup pot over medium-high, heat the olive oil until it shimmers.

2. Add the mustard seeds and cumin seeds to the pot, and cook for 30 seconds or just until the mustard seeds begin to pop. Add the onion and cook, stirring often, for 2 minutes or until the onion begins to soften. Add the cauliflower and reduce the heat to medium-low. Cook for 5 minutes, stirring often.

3. Add the curry powder, turmeric, cumin, and salt to the cauliflower mixture. Cook for 1 minute, stirring often. Stir in the broccoli and vegetable broth. Increase the heat to medium-high and bring the mixture to a boil. Reduce the heat and simmer for 5 minutes or until the broccoli is tender.

4. Stir in the coconut milk and cook for an additional 2 minutes or until the dal is heated through.

INGREDIENT TIP: To add a little heat to this soup, add ½ teaspoon cayenne pepper in step 3. For a more complex spiced flavor, substitute an equal amount of garam masala for the yellow curry powder.

PER SERVING (1½ CUPS): Calories: 252; Total fat: 20g; Total carbs: 13g; Fiber: 4.5g; Net carbs: 8.5g; Protein: 5g

Italian Wedding Soup

This one-pot soup is quick, easy, and studded with mini meatballs. Cauliflower rice subs in nicely for pasta.

FOR THE MEATBALLS

½ pound 80/20 ground beef

½ pound ground pork

½ cup grated Parmesan cheese

¼ cup diced yellow onion

1 large egg

2 garlic cloves, minced

1 teaspoon salt

½ teaspoon freshly ground black pepper

1 tablespoon extra-virgin olive oil

FOR THE SOUP

1 tablespoon extra-virgin olive oil

¼ cup chopped yellow onion

½ cup chopped celery

3 garlic cloves, minced

96 ounces (12 cups) reduced-sodium chicken broth

2 cups riced cauliflower

4 cups packed baby spinach leaves

¼ cup choppeddill weed

TO MAKE THE MEATBALLS

1. In a large bowl, combine the ground beef, ground pork, Parmesan, onion, egg, garlic, salt, and pepper. Mix well.

2. Measure out ½ tablespoon of the meat mixture and, using your hands, shape into a mini meatball. Repeat until all of the meat mixture has been used (you should have about 42 mini meatballs).

3. In a large soup pot over medium-high heat, heat the olive oil until it shimmers. Working in batches if needed, cook the meatballs for 5 minutes, turning periodically, until browned on all sides. Transfer the cooked meatballs to a plate. Wipe the pot clean with a paper towel and reserve.

TO MAKE THE SOUP

4. Using the clean pot over medium-high heat, heat the olive oil until it shimmers. Add the onion, celery, and garlic, and cook, stirring occasionally, for 2 minutes or until the vegetables start to soften.

5. Stir in the chicken broth and the cauliflower. Bring the mixture to a boil, and reduce the heat and simmer for 10 minutes, until the cauliflower is tender-crisp (it still has a little bite).

6. Stir in the spinach and dill, and cook for 2 minutes, just until the spinach has wilted.

7. Return the meatballs to the pot and cook for an additional 2 minutes, until the meatballs have warmed through.

VARIATION: Ground chicken, turkey, and sausage will all make delicious meatballs for your soup.

PER SERVING (2 CUPS + 7 MEATBALLS): Calories: 268; Total fat: 16g; Total carbs: 8g; Fiber: 2g; Net carbs: 6g; Protein: 23g

Egg and Olive Salad

SERVES: **3** | 5 Ingredients or Less, 30 Minutes or Less, Dairy-Free, One Pot, Quick Prep, Vegetarian
PREP TIME: **5 minutes**

This salad is excellent served in romaine lettuce leaves or a Cauliflower Tortilla, and makes a great lunch or simple snack to boost protein and fats (see here for how to perfectly boil eggs).

4 large hard-boiled eggs, coarsely chopped

⅓ cup sliced green olives

½ teaspoon salt

¼ teaspoon cayenne pepper

¼ cup keto-friendly mayonnaise or Avocado Oil Mayonnaise

1. In a medium bowl, combine the eggs, olives, salt, and cayenne pepper.

2. Add the mayonnaise and stir until creamy.

FLAVOR BOOST: For a zestier flavor, add 2 minced garlic cloves and 1 teaspoon horseradish or yellow mustard to the egg yolk mixture.

PER SERVING: Calories: 239; Total fat: 22g; Total carbs: 1.5g; Fiber: 0g; Net carbs: 1.5g; Protein: 8.5g

Garlic Shrimp, Asparagus, and Cilantro Salad

SERVES: 4 | 30 Minutes or Less, Dairy-Free, Quick Prep
PREP TIME: 10 minutes | COOK TIME: 5 minutes

If you're a cilantro lover like me, you'll love this salad. Freshness counts here: Look for cilantro that has crisp and vibrant stems and leaves. Pro tip: Use a potato peeler to thinly shave the asparagus spears.

3 tablespoons extra-virgin olive oil, divided

2 large garlic cloves, diced

16 ounces raw (36 to 40) large shrimp, shelled and deveined

1 large bunch fresh cilantro, roughly chopped

1 bunch asparagus spears, shaved

¼ cup thinly sliced red onion strips

1 teaspoon lime zest

2 tablespoons fresh lime juice

1 teaspoon powdered natural sweetener

½ teaspoon Dijon mustard

½ teaspoon salt

¼ teaspoon freshly ground black pepper

1. In a large skillet over medium-high heat, heat 1 tablespoon of olive oil until it shimmers. Add the garlic and cook, stirring constantly, for 30 seconds. Add the shrimp and cook for 2 minutes on each side, until the shrimp is no longer opaque. Transfer the cooked shrimp to a plate and set aside.

2. In a large salad bowl, combine the cilantro, shaved asparagus, and red onion. Toss to combine. Set aside.

3. In a small bowl, whisk together the remaining 2 tablespoons of olive oil, lime zest, lime juice, natural sweetener, mustard, salt, and pepper until well incorporated.

4. Pour the lime dressing over the shrimp and toss gently until well coated. Serve the dressed shrimp over the cilantro mixture.

SUBSTITUTION TIP: Pre-cooked thawed shrimp can be used in place of the raw shrimp. Make sure the shrimp has been patted dry with a paper towel. Add it to the olive oil mixture in step 3. Cook, stirring, for 30 seconds. Remove the cooked shrimp from the heat immediately and proceed with the recipe.

PER SERVING: Calories: 184; Total fat: 10g; Total carbs: 2.5g; Fiber: 1g; Net carbs: 1.5g; Protein: 21g

Keto Cobb Salad

SERVES: **4** | 30 Minutes or Less
PREP TIME: **15 minutes**

Rotisserie chicken makes this a quick lunch or light dinner. Serve this with the Cilantro Lime Vinaigrette or the Chipotle Ranch Dressing. If you prefer a store-bought dressing, G. Hughes makes a sugar-free keto-friendly Italian dressing that can be found in most grocery stores or online.

4 cups packed chopped romaine lettuce

2 cups packed chopped Boston lettuce

1 small bunch watercress

4 cups chopped cooked chicken breast

8 slices uncured, sugar-free cooked bacon, chopped

1 cup halved cherry tomatoes

2 avocados, pitted, peeled, and sliced

4 hard-boiled eggs, peeled and cut into quarters

½ cup crumbly full-fat blue cheese

¼ cup finely chopped fresh chives

½ cup salad dressing of choice

Salt

Freshly ground black pepper

1. In a large salad bowl, toss together the romaine lettuce, Boston lettuce, and watercress. Set aside.

2. On a large platter, arrange the chicken, bacon, tomatoes, and avocados in diagonal rows. Top with the quartered eggs, and sprinkle with blue cheese and chives.

3. To serve, divide the salad into four smaller salad bowls or plates. Top with a selection of chicken, bacon, tomatoes,

avocadoes, eggs, blue cheese, and chives, to taste. Drizzle with the salad dressing and sprinkle with salt and pepper (if using) just prior to serving.

VARIATION: Substitute an equal amount of cooked shrimp or turkey for the chicken breast. You can also sub in cubed cheddar or Monterey jack cheese for the blue cheese. You can also add sliced red onion to this salad for additional crunch and flavor.

PER SERVING: Calories: 597; Total fat: 41g; Total carbs: 13g; Fiber: 7g; Net carbs: 6g; Protein: 44g

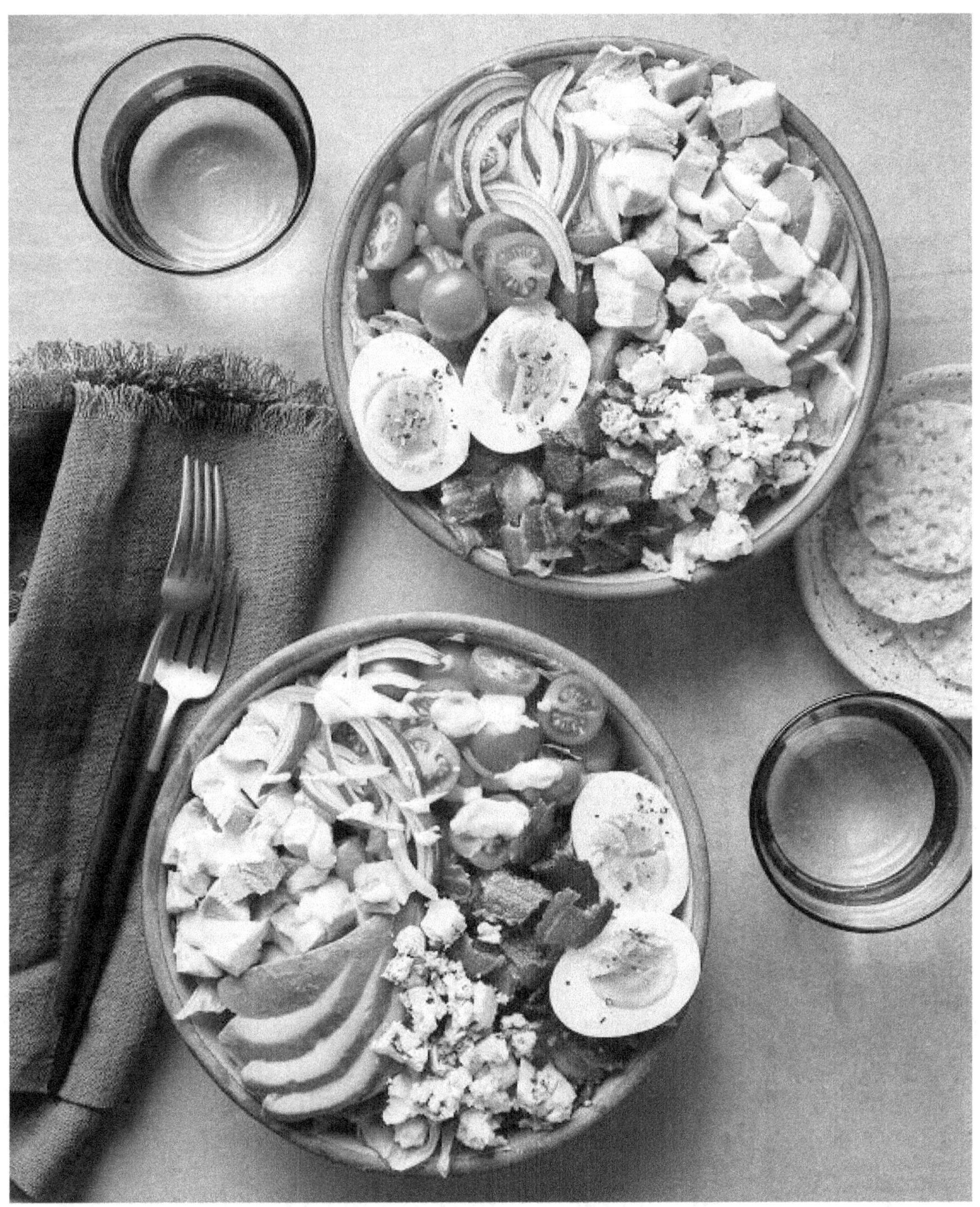

Roasted Cauliflower Salad

SERVES: 4 | 5 Ingredients or Less, 30 Minutes or Less, One Pot, Quick Prep, Vegetarian
PREP TIME: 5 minutes | COOK TIME: 25 minutes

Cauliflower is my favorite keto ingredient. I use it as a potato, pasta, and rice substitute in many recipes and am never disappointed. One medium head of cauliflower usually yields about 4 cups of florets. To save time, feel free to purchase pre-cut cauliflower.

4 cups cauliflower florets

2 tablespoons extra-virgin olive oil

½ teaspoon freshly ground black pepper, divided

1 cup grape tomatoes

1 cup full-fat feta cheese

1 cup pitted kalamata olives

1 tablespoon fresh lemon juice

1. Preheat the oven to 375°F.

2. Arrange the cauliflower florets in a single layer on a large baking sheet. Drizzle with the olive oil. Season with half the pepper. Roast for 25 minutes, turning once, until the cauliflower is caramelized around the edges and fork-tender.

3. Remove the pan from the oven and transfer the cooked cauliflower to a serving bowl. Add the tomatoes, feta, kalamata olives, lemon juice, and remaining pepper. Toss to combine. Serve warm or cold.

VARIATION: For a more colorful version with some zing, season the cauliflower with 1 teaspoon chili powder, ½ teaspoon ground cumin, ½ teaspoon salt, and ¼ teaspoon cayenne pepper in step 2. In step 3, substitute crumbled cotija cheese for the feta, and add 1 seeded and diced red bell pepper, 1 tablespoon fresh lime juice, and ½ cup fresh chopped fresh cilantro leaves.

PER SERVING: Calories: 218; Total fat: 17g; Total carbs: 7g; Fiber: 2g; Net carbs: 5g; Protein: 8g

Sweet and Spicy Broccoli Salad

Traditionally, broccoli salad includes raisins, which are not keto-friendly. I've replaced the raisins with diced red bell pepper along with a little powdered natural sweetener (to mimic the sweetness raisins would add). If you don't have precooked bacon bits on hand, I recommend cooking the bacon in the oven at 400°F for 15 minutes, turning halfway, or until you reach your desired crispness.

5 cups broccoli florets

½ medium red bell pepper, seeded and diced

1 jalapeño pepper, seeded and diced

3 scallions, green and white parts, diced

1 cup shredded full-fat cheddar cheese

8 slices cooked uncured, sugar-free bacon, crumbled

½ cup unsalted sunflower seeds

1 cup keto-friendly mayonnaise or Avocado Oil Mayonnaise

2 tablespoons apple cider vinegar

3 teaspoons powdered natural sweetener (optional)

1. In a large bowl, combine the broccoli, red bell pepper, jalapeño pepper, scallions, cheese, bacon, and sunflower seeds.

2. In a small bowl, whisk together the mayonnaise, vinegar, and natural sweetener (if using). Pour the mayonnaise mixture into the broccoli mixture and stir until well combined.

Steak Salad

SERVES: 4 | 5 Ingredients or Less, 30 Minutes or Less, One Pot, Quick Prep
PREP TIME: 5 minutes | COOK TIME: 12 minutes, plus 8 minutes to rest

This steak salad is super simple to make. The recipe calls for the steaks to be cooked to medium rare (130°F), which is just browned around the outer layer of the meat with a warm red center. Feel free to cook the steak to your own preferred level of doneness.

1 pound sirloin or skirt steak

1 teaspoon salt

½ teaspoon freshly ground black pepper

8 cups chopped romaine lettuce

1 avocado, peeled, pitted, and sliced

1 cup cherry tomatoes, sliced in half

½ cup crumbled full-fat blue cheese

1. Preheat a grill or grill pan over medium-high heat until hot.

2. Season the steak with the salt and pepper on both sides, being careful to apply the season evenly. Place the steak on the hot grill or grill pan and cook (without flipping) for 6 minutes. Turn the steak over and cook the other side for an additional 6 minutes or until the internal temperature indicates 130°F.

3. Transfer the steak to a cutting board, tent with foil, and let rest for 8 minutes. Using a serrated knife, cut the steak against the grain into ¼-inch slices.

4. To serve, place 2 cups of the lettuce on each of four salad plates and top with one-quarter each of the steak slices, avocado, and tomatoes. Top each serving with 2 tablespoons of crumbled blue cheese.

FLAVOR BOOST: Serve with 2 tablespoons of keto-friendly creamy blue cheese dressing or 2 tablespoons <u>Chipotle Ranch Dressing</u>.

PER SERVING: Calories: 315; Total fat: 18.5g; Total carbs: 7g; Fiber: 4.5g; Net carbs: 2.5g; Protein: 30g

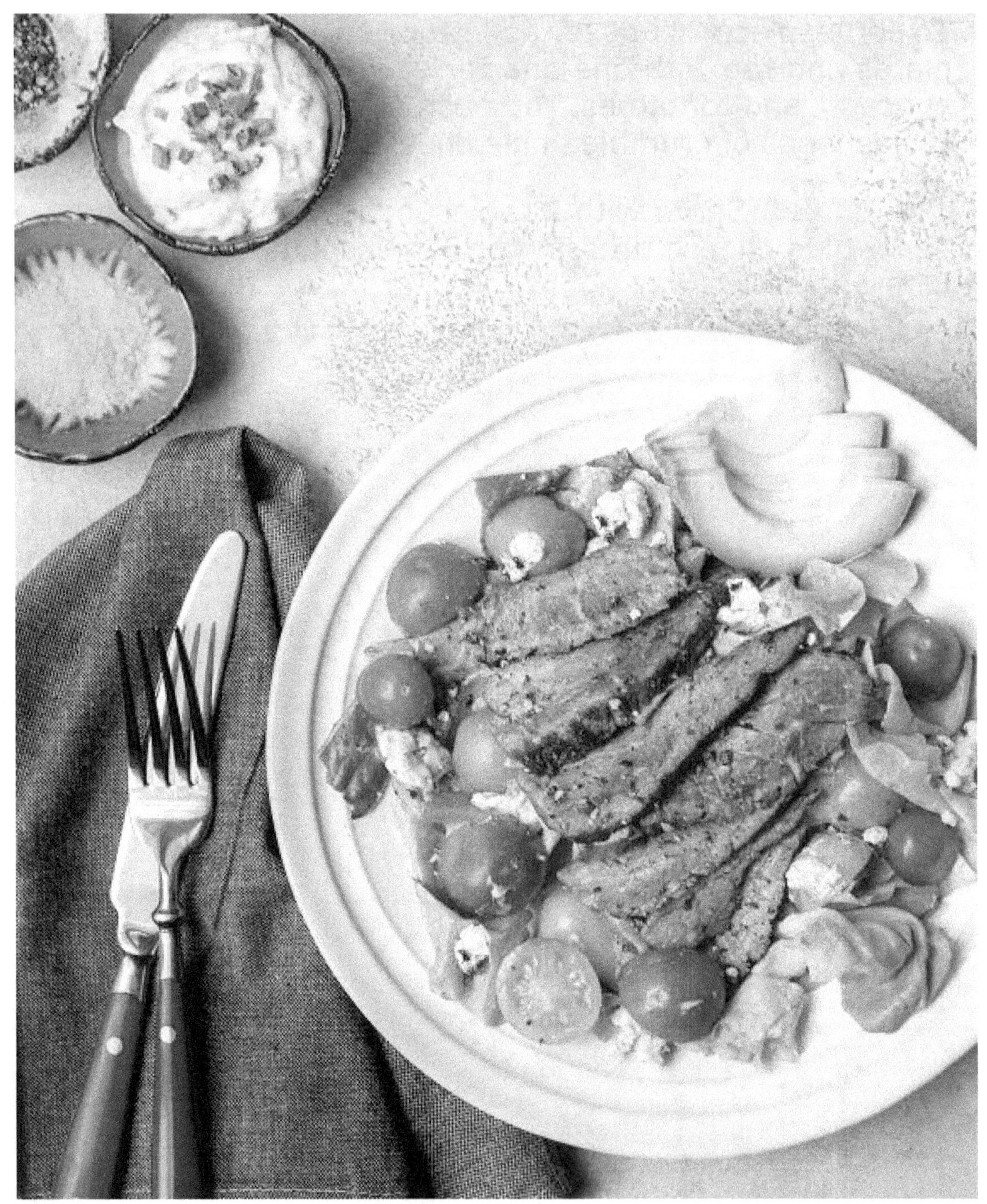

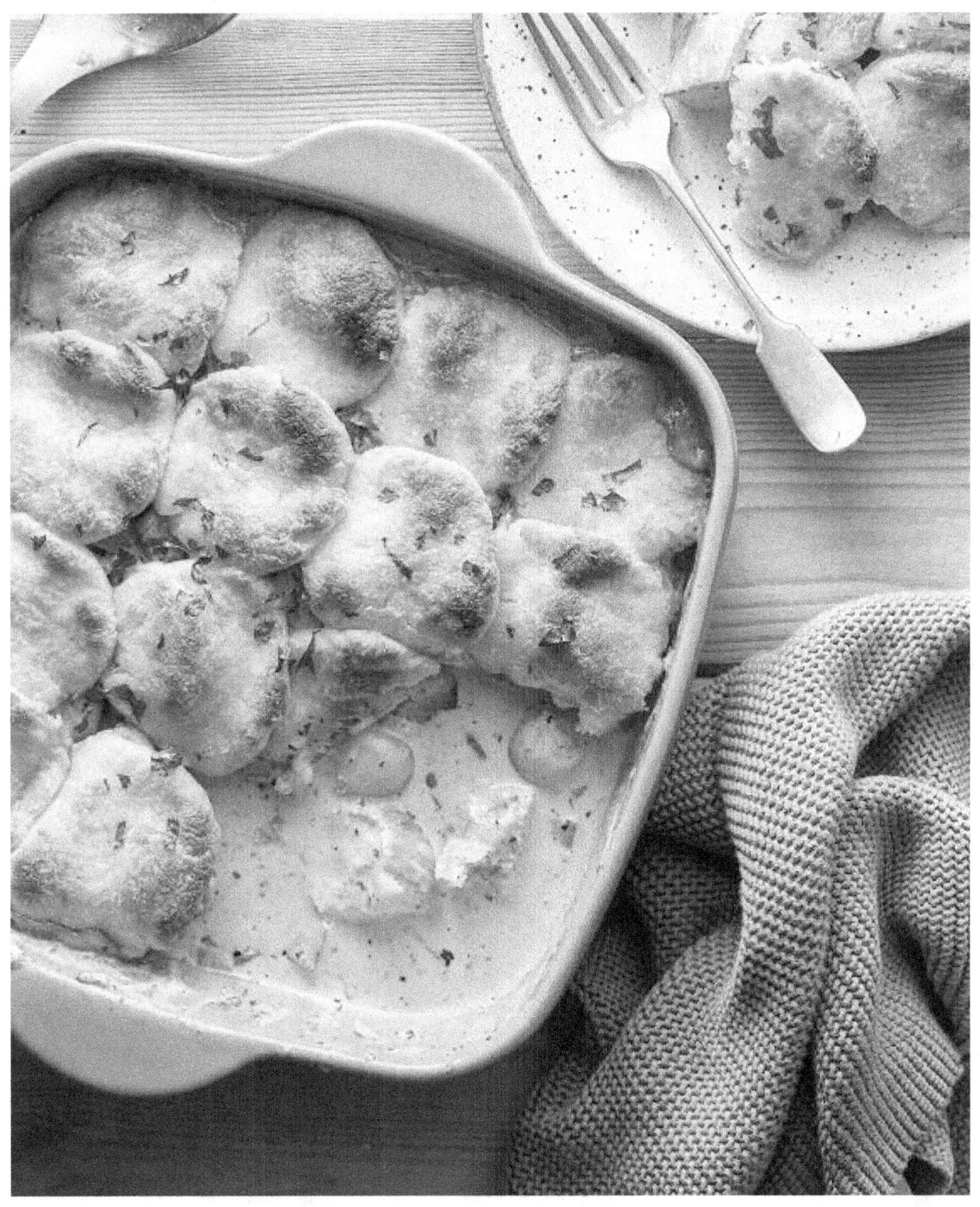

Chicken Pot Pie

6

Poultry and Seafood

Chicken Pot Pie
Cheesy-Stuffed Chicken with Spicy Sauce
Chicken Kebabs
Chicken Fajita Pizza
Keto Chicken Nuggets
Ground Turkey Stir-Fry
Shrimp with Zoodles
Creamy Fish Scampi
Keto Salmon Cakes
Shrimp Skewers
Maple-Garlic Salmon with Toasted Walnuts
Homemade Fish Sticks
Seared Scallops with Cilantro Lime Vinaigrette

CHicken Pot Pie

This version of chicken pot pie is pure keto comfort food, with cream cheese used as the thickening agent in the gravy. Be sure to use full-fat cream cheese and bring it to room temperature before using. Although carrots are considered a higher-carb vegetable, there are not enough of them in this recipe to cause a significant increase in carbs. Garnish with 1 tablespoon of fresh chopped parsley, if desired.

FOR THE FILLING

Olive oil cooking spray

2 tablespoons extra-virgin olive oil

2 pounds boneless, skinless chicken breasts, cut into 1-inch pieces

1 teaspoon salt

½ teaspoon freshly ground black pepper

1 cup chopped green beans

½ cup shredded carrots

½ cup diced yellow onion or ½ cup pearl onions

3 large garlic cloves

1 teaspoon minced fresh sage

1 teaspoon fresh thyme leaves

8 ounces full-fat cream cheese

1 cup reduced-sodium chicken broth

FOR THE BISCUITS

2 cups almond flour

2 tablespoons baking powder

1 teaspoon garlic powder

½ teaspoon salt

1½ cups shredded full-fat cheddar cheese

1 large egg, whisked

½ cup half and half

4 tablespoons unsalted butter, melted

TO MAKE THE FILLING

1. Preheat the oven to 350°F. Spray a large baking dish with cooking spray. Set aside.

2. In a large skillet over medium-high heat, heat the olive oil until it shimmers. Place the chicken in the hot skillet and season with the salt and pepper. Cook for 7 minutes, stirring occasionally, until the chicken is browned on all sides.

3. Add the green beans, carrots, onion, garlic, sage, and thyme to the skillet. Cook, stirring occasionally, for 7 minutes, until the beans are tender and the chicken is cooked through.

4. Add the cream cheese to the skillet and cook, stirring constantly, until the cream cheese is incorporated into the chicken mixture. Stir in the chicken broth, and simmer for 5 minutes.

5. Transfer the chicken mixture to the prepared baking dish. Set aside.

TO MAKE THE BISCUITS

6. In a large bowl, whisk together the almond flour, baking powder, garlic powder, and salt. Add the cheddar cheese and toss to coat.

7. Make a well in the center of the flour mixture. Add the egg, half and half, and melted butter. Stir until well incorporated. You should have a somewhat sticky dough.

8. Drop large tablespoon-size portions of dough on top of the chicken mixture in an even layer so the filling is completely covered.

9. Bake for 30 minutes or until the biscuits are golden on top and a toothpick inserted into the center of one comes out clean.

FLAVOR BOOST: **For a delicious buttery topping, combine 1 teaspoon garlic powder, ½ teaspoon dried parsley, and 2 tablespoons melted butter in a small bowl. Brush evenly on top of the baked biscuits at the end of step 9, once the baking dish is removed from the oven.**

PER SERVING: Calories: 778; Total fat: 59g; Total carbs: 14g; Fiber: 5g; Net carbs: 9g; Protein: 49g

Cheesy-Stuffed Chicken with Spicy Sauce

SERVES: 4 | Worth the Wait
PREP TIME: 15 minutes | COOK TIME: 20 minutes

These stuffed chicken breasts are a delicious, healthier alternative to fried chicken wings (and deliver a bigger serving size as well). To give that hot wing feel, I drizzle them with hot sauce. I love to serve these with a side of steamed broccoli or Glazed Mushrooms.

⅔ cup full-fat blue cheese

1 tablespoon full-fat sour cream

1 teaspoon fresh lemon juice

⅛ teaspoon freshly ground black pepper

4 (6-ounce) boneless, skinless chicken breasts

¼ cup coconut flour

¾ cup almond flour

1 large egg

2 tablespoons heavy (whipping) cream

2 tablespoons hot sauce, divided

3 tablespoons unsalted butter, divided

1 teaspoon coconut aminos

1 garlic clove, minced

1. Preheat the oven to 350°F.

2. In a small bowl, combine the blue cheese, sour cream, lemon juice, and black pepper. Stir well, and then set aside.

3. Using a sharp knife, cut a horizontal slit in each chicken breast to form a pocket. Divide the cheese mixture into

four even portions, and stuff each portion into the chicken pockets. Set aside.

4. Place the coconut flour in a shallow dish. Place the almond flour in another shallow dish. In a third shallow dish, whisk the egg with the heavy cream and 1 tablespoon of the hot sauce.

5. Working with 1 chicken breast half at a time, dredge the chicken first in the coconut flour, and then in the egg mixture, and then in the almond flour, being careful to ensure each breast is coated completely in each step.

6. Heat a large ovenproof skillet over medium-high heat. Place 1 tablespoon of the butter in the hot pan and swirl until the butter melts. Arrange the stuffed chicken breasts in the skillet and cook on one side for 4 minutes or until browned. Carefully turn the chicken over, and then place the skillet in the preheated oven. Bake for 20 minutes, or until the chicken is cooked through (reaches an internal temperature of 160°F).

7. Meanwhile, in a small saucepan, combine the remaining 2 tablespoons of the butter, coconut aminos, and garlic. Warm over medium heat until the butter has completely melted. Remove from the heat and stir in the remaining 1 tablespoon of the hot sauce. Evenly distribute the sauce over the chicken when serving.

VARIATION: Omit the almond flour coating by skipping this part of the instructions in steps 4 and 5.

PER SERVING: Calories: 479; Total fat: 30.5g; Total carbs: 7g; Fiber: 4g; Net carbs: 3g; Protein: 44g

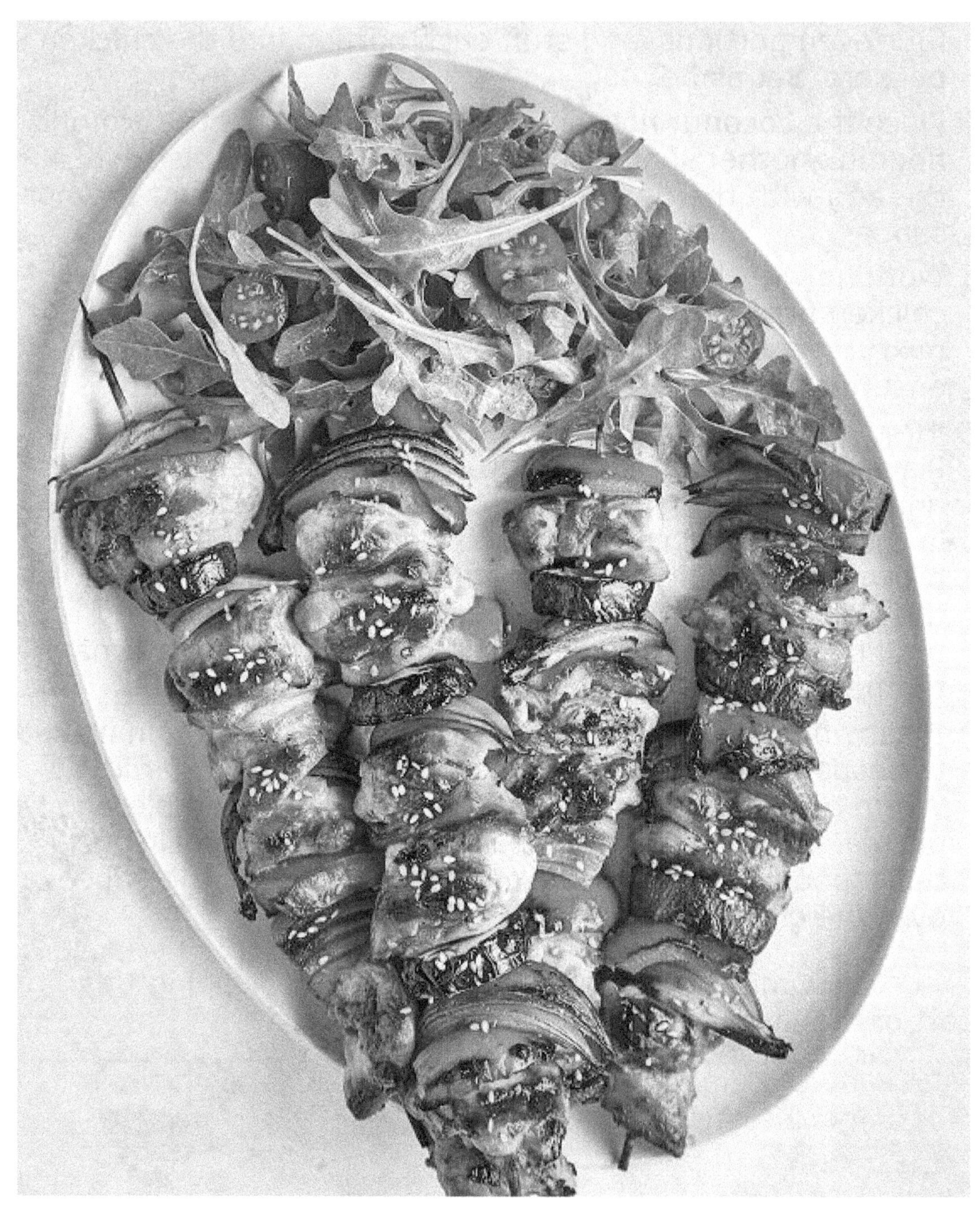

CHicken Kebabs

These chicken kebabs are great on their own or served alongside Creamy Coleslaw, Cauliflower Fried Rice, or a simple arugula salad. Try to keep the vegetables and chicken pieces as uniform in size as possible, approximately ¾- to 1-inch thick. Soak the wooden skewers for 30 minutes before assembling to prevent the skewers from burning during grilling.

1 pound boneless, skinless chicken thighs, cubed

¼ cup coconut aminos

¼ cup extra-virgin olive oil

¼ cup fresh lemon juice

4 large garlic cloves, minced

1 tablespoon brown sugar natural sweetener (optional)

1 teaspoon salt

½ teaspoon freshly ground black pepper

2 small zucchinis, sliced

1 red bell pepper, seeded and cubed

1 red onion, cubed

1 teaspoon toasted sesame seeds (optional)

1. In a large bowl with a lid or in a large resealable bag, combine the chicken, coconut aminos, olive oil, lemon juice, garlic, natural sweetener (if using), salt, and black pepper. Seal and then toss until well coated. Refrigerate for 30 minutes.

2. Preheat the grill to medium-high.

3. Thread the wooden skewers with alternating pieces of chicken and the zucchini, red pepper, and red onion, leaving ¼ inch of space between each piece to allow for even heat distribution. Grill the kebabs, turning occasionally, for 13 minutes or until the chicken is cooked through (internal temperature reaches 165°F) and the vegetables are crisp-tender.

4. Transfer the kebabs to a serving dish and sprinkle with toasted sesame seeds (if using).

VARIATION: Use any combination of eggplant, yellow squash, and button mushrooms in place of the zucchini, bell pepper, and onion.

PER SERVING: Calories: 309; Total fat: 20.5g; Total carbs: 10g; Fiber: 1.5g; Net carbs: 8.5g; Protein: 21g

Chicken Fajita Pizza

SERVES: **4** | 30 Minutes or Less, Quick Prep
PREP TIME: **10 minutes** | COOK TIME: **20 minutes**

The Chicken Pizza Crust provides all the protein you need in this dish. And it's so versatile, you can use it to make any type of pizza you desire. This chicken fajita pizza is a great place to start. Make sure the salsa you choose is keto-friendly (no sugar added).

1 tablespoon extra-virgin olive oil

1 cup sliced yellow onion

1 cup sliced red bell pepper

1 cup sliced green bell pepper

1 teaspoon chili powder

1 teaspoon ground cumin

½ teaspoon garlic powder

1 pre-cooked Chicken Pizza Crust

½ cup keto-friendly salsa (I like Frontera brand)

1 cup part-skim shredded mozzarella

1 cup shredded full-fat Colby jack cheese

¼ cup chopped fresh cilantro

½ cup full-fat sour cream (optional)

1. Preheat the oven to 350°F. Line a baking sheet with parchment paper and set aside.

2. In a large skillet over medium-high heat, heat the olive oil until it shimmers. Add the onion, red pepper, and green pepper. Cook for 3 minutes, or until the vegetables are crisp-tender. Stir in the chili powder, cumin, and garlic powder. Remove the pan from the heat and set aside.

3. Place the chicken pizza crust on the prepared baking sheet. Spread the salsa evenly over the crust. Sprinkle the salsa with the mozzarella cheese and Colby jack cheese. Top with the pepper mixture. Bake for 20 minutes or until the cheese has melted and browned around the edges.

4. Remove the pan from the oven. Sprinkle the pizza with the cilantro. Cut into wedges and serve with sour cream (if using).

FLAVOR BOOST: For a little heat, add 1 sliced jalapeño pepper to the pan in step 2, along with the bell peppers and onion.

PER SERVING: Calories: 276; Total fat: 18g; Total carbs: 6g; Fiber: 1g; Net carbs: 5g; Protein: 25g

Keto Chicken Nuggets

Using canned chicken to make these fan favorites allows the seasoning to permeate throughout the nugget, but you can also use any leftover chicken or turkey you have on hand. Serve these nuggets with Fry Dipping Sauce or Chipotle Ranch Dressing.

Olive oil cooking spray

12.5 ounces canned chicken, drained

¾ cup almond flour, divided

1 large egg

1 cup part-skim shredded mozzarella cheese

1 teaspoon onion powder

1 teaspoon garlic powder

1. Preheat the oven to 400°F. Lightly coat a baking sheet with cooking spray and set aside.

2. In a large bowl, combine the chicken, ½ cup of the almond flour, egg, cheese, onion powder, and garlic powder. Mix until all the ingredients are well incorporated.

3. Place the remaining ¼ cup almond flour in a shallow bowl. Using a small cookie scoop or tablespoon, scoop out a portion of the chicken mixture and, using your hands, shape it into a nugget. Place the nugget on a plate, and repeat with the remaining mixture to make 18 nuggets.

4. Roll each chicken nugget in the almond flour mixture, coating all sides. Place the coated nuggets on the prepared baking sheet.

5. Bake for 8 minutes, or until the bottom of the chicken nuggets are crispy. Flip the chicken nuggets and bake for an additional 7 minutes, or until browned and cooked through (reaches an internal temperature of 160°F).

PER SERVING (6 NUGGETS): Calories: 415; Total fat: 25g; Total Carbs: 9g; Fiber: 3g; Net carbs: 6g; Protein 38g

Ground Turkey Stir-Fry

SERVES: **4** | 30 Minutes or Less, Dairy-Free, One Pot, Quick Prep
PREP TIME: **10 minutes** | COOK TIME: **15 minutes**

If you like Asian fusion, you'll love this ground turkey stir-fry. Full of scallions, garlic, ginger, and cabbage (keto-friendly veggies), its flavor will remind you of your favorite eggroll. I like to buy ginger paste in a tube because I find it lasts longer and is easier to use. Look for it in the produce section of the grocery store where you find the fresh herbs.

1 tablespoon extra-virgin olive oil

2 scallions, sliced, white and green parts separated

2 large garlic cloves, minced

1 teaspoon ginger paste

1 pound ground turkey

4 cups shredded cabbage (red, white, or a combination of both)

2 tablespoons coconut aminos

1 tablespoon unseasoned rice vinegar

4 teaspoons sriracha sauce (optional)

1 teaspoon toasted sesame seeds (optional)

1. In a large skillet over medium heat, heat the oil until it shimmers. Add the scallions, garlic, and ginger. Cook, stirring, for 1 minute, until the garlic is fragrant.

2. Crumble in the ground turkey. Using a wooden spoon, break the meat into smaller pieces and cook, stirring often, for 8 minutes or just until the turkey begins to brown.

3. Add the cabbage, coconut aminos, and rice vinegar to the turkey mixture. Cook for 8 minutes, until the cabbage is tender and wilted and the ground meat is fully browned and cooked through.

4. Serve with sriracha sauce and toasted sesame seeds (if using).

VARIATION: Save time by purchasing pre-shredded cabbage. Use ground beef, pork, chicken, or sweet sausage in place of the ground turkey.

PER SERVING: Calories: 227; Total fat: 12g; Total carbs: 6.5g; Fiber: 2g; Net carbs: 4.5g; Protein: 23g

Shrimp with Zoodles

SERVES: **4** | 5 Ingredients or Less, 30 Minutes or Less, One Pot

PREP TIME: **15 minutes** | COOK TIME: **15 minutes**

This is a super-fast and easy dinner to get on the table on busy nights. You can buy the zucchini already spiralized or make it yourself. Just remember: the longer you cook the zoodles, the mushier they will get, so keep a close eye on them when cooking.

1 tablespoon extra-virgin olive oil, divided

4 garlic cloves, minced

16 ounces large (36 to 40) raw shrimp peeled and deveined

1 teaspoon salt

½ teaspoon freshly ground black pepper

1 tablespoon fresh lemon juice

2 small zucchini, spiralized, or 6 cups zucchini noodles

2 tablespoons grated Parmesan cheese

1 tablespoon minced fresh parsley leaves

1. In a large skillet over medium-high heat, heat ½ tablespoon of the olive oil until it shimmers. Add the garlic and cook for 30 seconds, until fragrant but not brown.

2. Add the shrimp to the skillet and season with the salt and pepper. Cook for 2 minutes on each side, or until the shrimp is opaque and cooked through. Remove the pan from the heat.

3. Drizzle the lemon juice over the shrimp and gently toss until coated. Transfer the cooked shrimp to a plate, reserving the skillet, and set aside.

4. Add the spiralized zucchini and the remaining ½ tablespoon of olive oil to the reserved skillet. Cook over medium-high heat for 3 minutes, tossing often (use tongs, if it helps). Transfer the cooked zoodles to a large serving bowl. Top with the shrimp. Sprinkle with the Parmesan and parsley. Serve immediately.

INGREDIENT TIP: This dish works equally well with a variety of spiralized vegetables: try substituting an equal amount of spiralized yellow squash, cucumber, broccoli stems, or radishes.

PER SERVING: Calories: 151; Total fat: 5g; Total carbs: 3g; Fiber: 0.5g; Net carbs: 2.5g; Protein: 24g

Creamy Fish Scampi

Cod, a mild, firm white fish that cooks quickly, is an excellent fish to eat on keto. It's high in protein and nutrients. This dish delivers all the flavors of your favorite shrimp scampi at a much more affordable price. If using frozen fillets, be sure to thaw them completely and then pat them dry with a paper towel to remove excess moisture prior to cooking. Serve with a side of Cauliflower Fried Rice.

1 tablespoon extra-virgin olive oil

2 garlic cloves, chopped fine

1 pound cod fish, cut into bite-size pieces

1 teaspoon salt

½ teaspoon freshly ground black pepper

¼ cup reduced-sodium chicken broth

¼ cup heavy (whipping) cream

1 teaspoon lemon zest

1 tablespoon fresh lemon juice

1 tablespoon chopped fresh parsley leaves

1. In a large skillet over medium-high heat, heat the olive oil until it shimmers. Add the garlic and fry for 30 seconds, until fragrant but not brown.

2. Add the cod, salt, and pepper to the skillet, and cook for 4 minutes, turning the fish occasionally, until the cod begins to flake but is still firm. Transfer the cooked cod to a plate, reserving the skillet, and set aside.

3. In the reserved skillet, combine the chicken broth, heavy cream, lemon zest, and lemon juice. Bring the broth mixture to a boil, reduce the heat, and simmer for 2 minutes or until the broth mixture has thickened.

4. Remove the skillet from the heat. Place the cooked cod pieces in the cream sauce and gently stir until the fish is well coated. Garnish with the parsley and serve immediately.

SUBSTITUTION TIP: Substitute any firm white fish, shrimp, or bay scallops for the cod fish.

PER SERVING: Calories: 211; Total fat: 14.5g; Total carbs: 1g; Fiber: 0g; Net carbs: 1g; Protein: 19g

Keto Salmon Cakes

Quick, easy, and satisfying, these salmon cakes are my go-to when I am in a pinch for time and need to get dinner on the table. When choosing canned salmon for this dish, quality matters. Check the label to make sure the salmon is wild caught and not farmed. My favorite brand is Wild Planet Wild Sockeye Salmon, and it can be found at Whole Foods Market or on Amazon.

20 ounces canned boneless, skinless salmon, drained

½ cup almond flour

2 large eggs

4 tablespoons finely minced red onion

2 tablespoons keto-friendly mayonnaise or Avocado Oil Mayonnaise

1 medium jalapeño pepper, diced fine (optional)

1 tablespoon chopped fresh cilantro leaves

½ teaspoon salt

¼ teaspoon freshly ground black pepper

4 tablespoons extra-virgin olive oil

1. In a large bowl, stir together the salmon, almond flour, eggs, red onion, mayonnaise, jalapeño (if using), cilantro, salt, and pepper.

2. Using ¼ cup measure and your hands, shape the salmon mixture into 8 patties.

3. In a skillet over medium–high heat, heat the oil until it shimmers. Working in batches so as not to crowd the pan,

fry the patties for 4 minutes on each side or until golden brown.

VARIATION: **Substitute a red or green bell pepper for the jalapeño pepper and/or canned tuna for the salmon.**

PER SERVING (2 SALMON CAKES): Calories: 399; Total fat: 27g; Total carbs: 3g; Fiber: 1.5g; Net carbs: 1.5g; Protein: 36g

Sнrimp Skewers

Shrimp is very low in carbs and is a great source of protein. Add Cauliflower Fried Rice, and you've got a complete meal. Or serve these skewers as an easy appetizer with a side of Fry Dipping Sauce or Cilantro Lime Vinaigrette for dipping.

1½ pounds raw large shrimp, tails on

¼ cup extra-virgin olive oil

1 teaspoon garlic powder

1 teaspoon smoked paprika

½ teaspoon ground cumin

½ teaspoon salt

¼ teaspoon freshly ground black pepper

1 recipe Cauliflower Fried Rice; optional)

1 tablespoon fresh lime juice (optional)

½ cup chopped fresh cilantro leaves (optional)

1. In a large bowl, toss the shrimp with the olive oil until well coated. Season with the garlic powder, paprika cumin, salt, and pepper, and toss again.

2. Heat a grill or grill pan over medium-high heat until hot.

3. Divide the shrimp into four equal servings and thread the shrimp evenly onto each of four skewers. Place the skewers on the grill. Cook for 2 minutes on each side, until the shrimp are opaque and cooked through.

4. Meanwhile, reheat the cauliflower fried rice (if using). Stir in the lime juice and cilantro (if using).

5. Serve the shrimp skewers over the cauliflower fried rice.

PER SERVING: Calories: 245; Total fat: 14g; Total carbs: 0g; Fiber: 0g; Net carbs: 0g; Protein: 30g

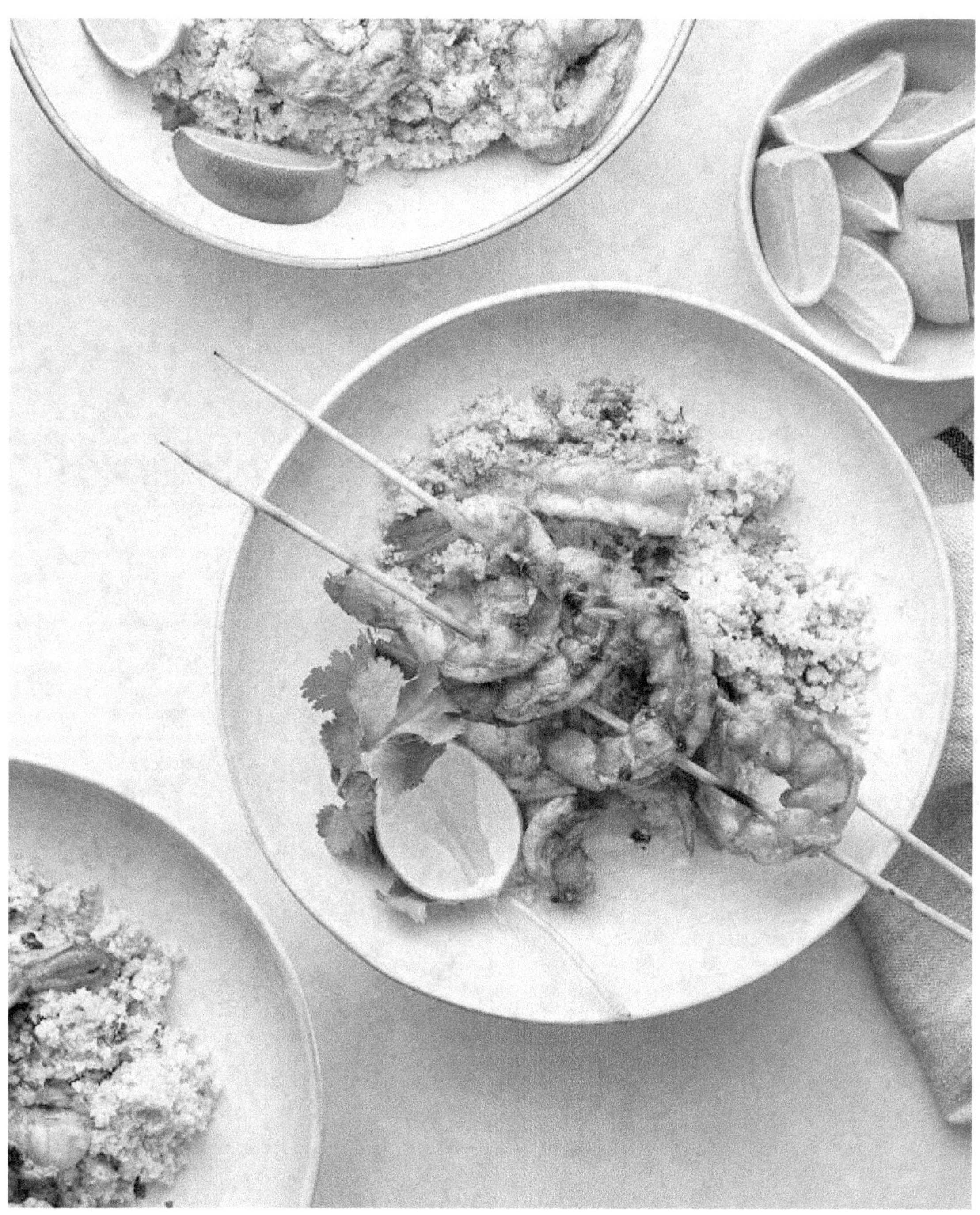

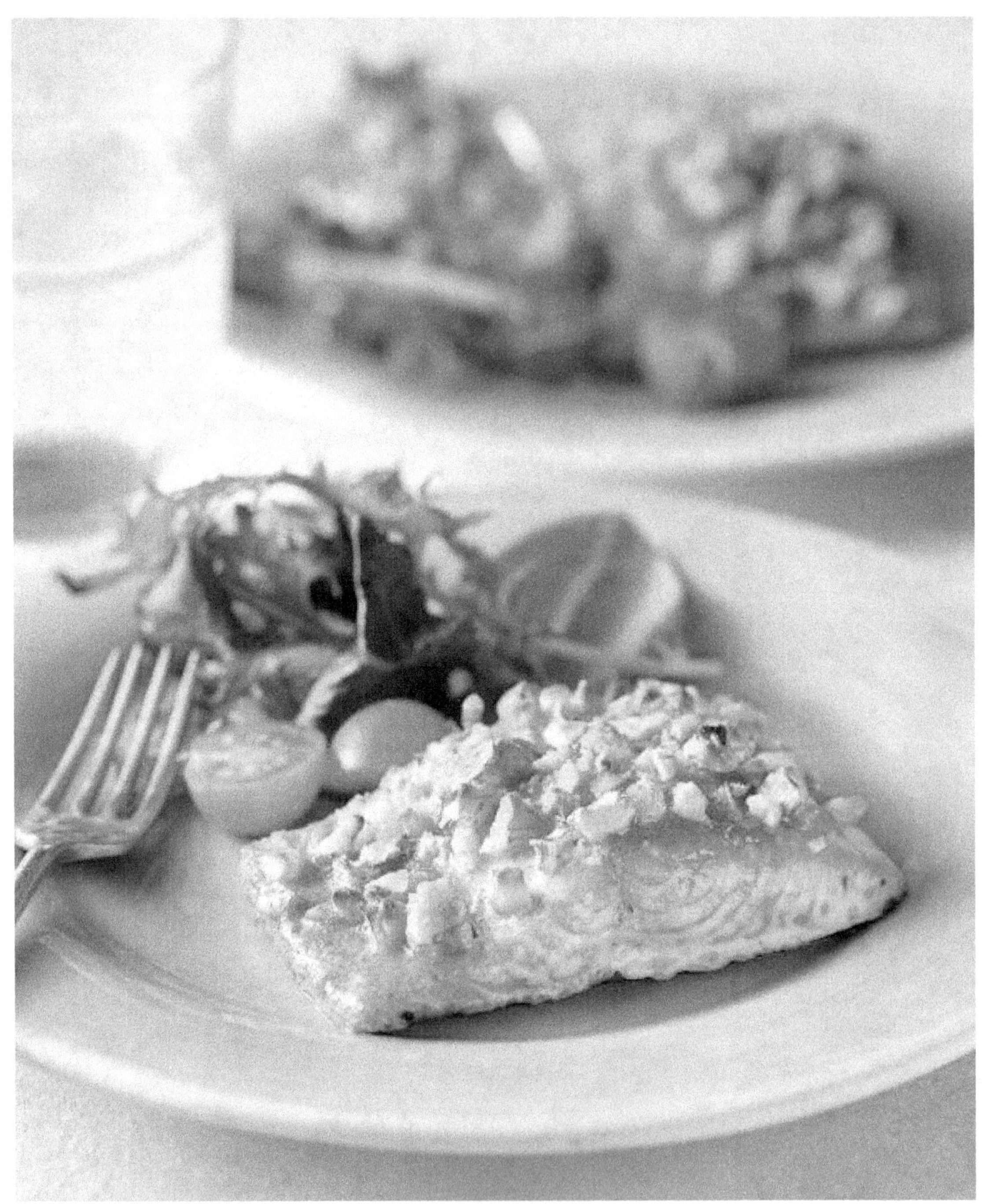

Maple-Garlic Salmon with Toasted Walnuts

SERVES: 4 | 30 Minutes or Less, Dairy-Free, Quick Prep
PREP TIME: 5 minutes | COOK TIME: 15 minutes

Salmon is packed with healthy fats and is one of the easiest proteins to prepare. Toasted walnuts add crunch to the maple-glazed fish. Depending on the thickness of your fillet, the cook time could be more or less, so watch carefully and begin checking for doneness after 12 minutes of cooking. Then remove the fish from the pan as soon as it's cooked through.

4 (4-ounce) salmon fillets

4 tablespoons Keto Maple Syrup, divided

1 teaspoon salt

½ teaspoon freshly ground black pepper

½ cup chopped walnuts

1 tablespoon Dijon mustard

½ teaspoon onion powder

½ teaspoon smoked paprika

1 tablespoon fresh chopped parsley leaves (optional)

1. Preheat the oven to 400°F. Line a large baking sheet with parchment paper.

2. Arrange the salmon fillets in a single layer on the prepared baking sheet. Drizzle each fillet with ½ tablespoon of maple syrup. Season with salt and pepper. Set aside.

3. In a small bowl, stir together the remaining 2 tablespoons of maple syrup, walnuts, mustard, onion powder, and paprika.

4. Spoon 2 tablespoons of the walnut mixture over each piece of salmon. Bake for 15 minutes or until the salmon is cooked through (opaque and flakes easily with a fork). Garnish with parsley (if using) and serve.

INGREDIENT TIP: Traditional maple syrup is not keto-friendly—it's predominantly sugar and, per tablespoon, contains as many carbs as you're allowed in a day—so be sure to make your own keto-friendly syrup or look for a similar product at the grocery store.

PER SERVING: Calories: 283; Total fat: 18g; Total carbs: 2g; Fiber: 1g; Net carbs: 1g; Protein: 28g

Homemade Fish Sticks

These fish sticks are crispy and low-carb thanks to the combo of almond flour and Parmesan in the crust. Shallow frying them in a pan with just enough oil to coat half the fish stick is a great alternative to deep-frying.

1 pound fresh cod fish fillet

1 large egg

½ cup almond flour

4 tablespoons grated Parmesan cheese

½ teaspoon garlic powder

½ teaspoon Old Bay seasoning (optional)

½ teaspoon salt

½ teaspoon freshly ground black pepper

2 cups extra-virgin olive oil (approx.), for frying

1. Using a sharp knife, cut the cod fillet into 2-inch-long pieces, 1-to-1½ inches thick. Set aside.

2. In a shallow bowl, whisk the egg until foamy. In another shallow bowl, combine the almond flour, Parmesan, garlic powder, Old Bay (if using), salt, and pepper.

3. Prepare your pan for frying: Pour about 2 inches deep of oil into a deep skillet. Heat over medium-high until the oil reaches 350°F or until a test piece of breaded fish sizzles when dropped into the hot oil.

4. Dip the fish pieces in the egg wash, and then dredge in the almond flour mixture, being careful to coat each piece

of fish completely. Place the breaded fish sticks on a parchment-lined baking sheet.

5. Working in batches so as not to crowd the pan, fry the fish sticks for 2 minutes on each side or until golden brown. Using tongs, transfer the fish sticks to a plate lined with paper towel to drain any excess oil. Keep warm until ready to serve.

PER SERVING: Calories: 323; Total fat: 25g; Total carbs: 2.5g; Fiber: 1g; Net carbs: 1.5g; Protein: 22g

Seared Scallops with Cilantro Lime Vinaigrette

SERVES: **4** | 5 Ingredients or Less, 30 Minutes or Less, Dairy-Free, One Pot, Quick Prep
PREP TIME: **5 minutes** | COOK TIME: **5 minutes**

These scallops develop a delicious, caramelized crust when cooking. Look for dry scallops, which are darker in color and have not been treated with any chemicals or additives. When preparing the scallops, pat them dry with paper towels to get the best sear possible.

1 pound dry sea scallops

1 teaspoon salt

½ teaspoon freshly ground black pepper

1 tablespoon extra-virgin olive oil

4 tablespoons Cilantro Lime Vinaigrette

1. Preheat a cast-iron skillet over medium-high heat.
2. Season the scallops with the salt and pepper.
3. Heat the oil in the skillet. Gently place the scallops in the skillet, leaving enough space between the scallops to allow steam to escape. Cook for 2 minutes, not moving or touching them. Using tongs, flip the scallops over and cook for 1 minute, until opaque and the bottom is browned.
4. Serve topped with the vinagrette.

FLAVOR BOOST: A cast-iron (rather than nonstick) skillet will deliver the best sear and caramelized crust possible.

PER SERVING: Calories: 171; Total fat: 11g; Total carbs: 4g; Fiber: 0g; Net carbs: 4g; Protein: 14g

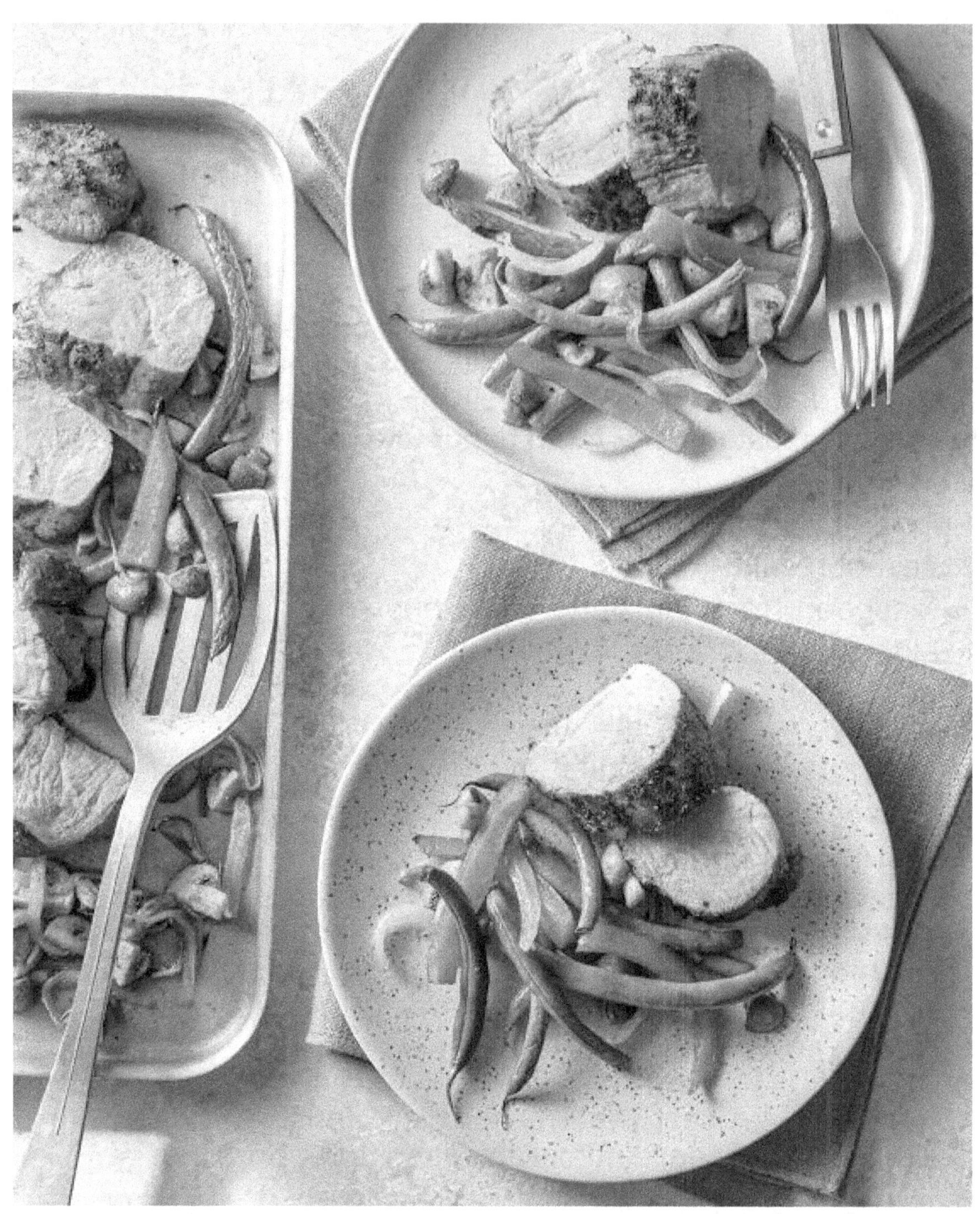

Sheet Pan Pork Tenderloin with Veggies

7

Pork and Beef

Pulled Pork
Sheet Pan Pork Tenderloin with Veggies
Dry Rub Ribs
Pork Chops
Beef and Broccoli Stir-Fry
Beef Burrito Bowl
Beef Tips with Creamy Mushroom Sauce
Sweet and Sour Meatloaf
Keto Shepherd's Pie
Breakfast for Dinner Burger Bowl
Keto Cabbage Roll Casserole
Ginger Garlic Pork Meatballs

Pulled Pork

SERVES: **8** | 5 Ingredients or Less, Dairy-Free, Worth the Wait
PREP TIME: **15 minutes** | COOK TIME: **6 hours**

You'll need your slow cooker for this pulled pork, which is very low in carbs and can be served on a keto-friendly roll, wrapped in lettuce and topped with sliced radishes and scallions, or in a Cauliflower Tortilla. It's excellent served with Creamy Coleslaw as either a topping or side. You can also make this ahead and use in Pulled Pork–Stuffed Mushrooms.

2 tablespoons yellow mustard

4 pounds pork shoulder roast

1 tablespoon chili powder

1 teaspoon ground cumin

1 tablespoon brown sugar natural sweetener

1 teaspoon salt

1 teaspoon freshly ground black pepper

⅓ cup water

1. Spread the mustard all over the roast. Place the roast in the slow cooker and set aside.

2. In a small bowl, combine the chili powder, cumin, natural sweetener, salt, and pepper. Sprinkle the mixture evenly over the roast.

3. Pour the water into the slow cooker, being careful not to pour it over the seasoned pork. Cover the slow cooker with the lid, and cook on low for 8 hours.

4. Transfer the pork to a platter, reserving the juices in the slow cooker. Using two forks, shred the meat.

5. Return the shredded meat to the slow cooker, and, using
   tongs, toss the meat in the juices until well coated.

COOKING TIP: To cook this recipe in an Instant Pot, pour the water in the bottom of the Instant Pot, and then add the pork loin. Cover with the lid and lock the release valve. Cook on manual high for 1 hour. When finished, do a natural release for 20 minutes. Proceed as directed in step 5.

PER SERVING: Calories: 430; Total fat: 28g; Total carbs: 1.5g; Fiber: 0g; Net carbs: 1.5g; Protein: 43g

Sheet Pan Pork Tenderloin with Veggies

SERVES: 6 | Dairy-Free, Quick Prep
PREP TIME: 10 minutes | COOK TIME: 30 minutes

This is a super-simple, fast, and delicious sheet pan meal. I like to reserve 1 teaspoon of the rub in step 2 to sprinkle over the veggies on the sheet pan, which adds flavor to every part of the meal.

2 tablespoons extra-virgin olive oil, divided

1 teaspoon ground cumin

1 teaspoon smoked paprika

1 teaspoon garlic powder

1 teaspoon salt

½ teaspoon freshly ground black pepper

2 pounds pork tenderloin

8 ounces button mushrooms, quartered

8 ounces green beans, trimmed

1 red bell pepper, cored, seeded, and sliced

1 large yellow onion, sliced

1. Preheat the oven to 425°F. Lightly grease a large baking sheet with 1 tablespoon of the olive oil and set aside.

2. In a small bowl, combine the cumin, paprika, garlic powder, salt, and black pepper. Reserve ½ teaspoon of the seasoning and set aside.

3. Place the pork tenderloin in the center of the prepared sheet pan. Using your hands, rub the remaining 1 tablespoon of the olive oil all over the pork. Sprinkle the seasoning mixture over the pork and, using your hands, rub the seasoning into the meat.

4. Arrange the mushrooms, green beans, bell pepper, and onion around the pork. Sprinkle the vegetables with the reserved seasoning mixture. Roast for 30 minutes or until the internal temperature of the pork reaches 165°F.

INGREDIENT TIP: To clean the mushrooms, simply wipe them off with a damp paper towel (never immerse mushrooms in water or they will become slimy). If the mushrooms are large, cut them into quarters; smaller mushrooms can be cut in half.

PER SERVING: Calories: 236; Total fat: 9g; Total carbs: 7g; Fiber: 2g; Net carbs: 5g; Protein: 32g

Dry Rub Ribs

SERVES: 6 | Dairy-Free, Quick Prep, Worth the Wait
PREP TIME: 5 minutes | COOK TIME: 2 hours 30 minutes

A long, slow bake time produces the most delicious, tender, and juicy ribs with a crisp exterior. The mustard coating adds flavor while preventing the seasoning from falling off the meat while cooking. These are delicious served with a side of Creamy Coleslaw and sprinkled with chopped chives.

2 tablespoons smoked paprika

1 tablespoon garlic powder

1 tablespoon onion powder

1 tablespoon chipotle powder

1½ teaspoons ground cumin

3 tablespoons brown sugar natural sweetener

½ cup spicy brown mustard

3 pounds pork ribs

1. Preheat the oven to 300°F. Line a baking sheet with aluminum foil and set aside.

2. In a small bowl, combine the paprika, garlic powder, onion powder, chipotle powder, cumin, and brown sugar natural sweetener.

3. Using your hands, spread the mustard evenly over both the top and back of the ribs. Then rub the spice mixture over the ribs, working it in fully and evenly.

4. Place the ribs on the prepared baking sheet. Bake for 2½ hours, or until the ribs are tender on the inside and crispy on the outside.

 Alternatively, cook these ribs on the grill over medium-high, indirect heat. Once the grill is preheated, turn off the burners on one side of the grill and place the ribs on the side where the burner has been turned off. Cook, turning every 30 minutes, for 3 hours, or until a light crust has formed and the internal temperature of the ribs reaches 145°F

PER SERVING: Calories: 303; Total fat: 23g; Total carbs: 0g; Fiber: 0g; Net carbs: 0g; Protein: 24g

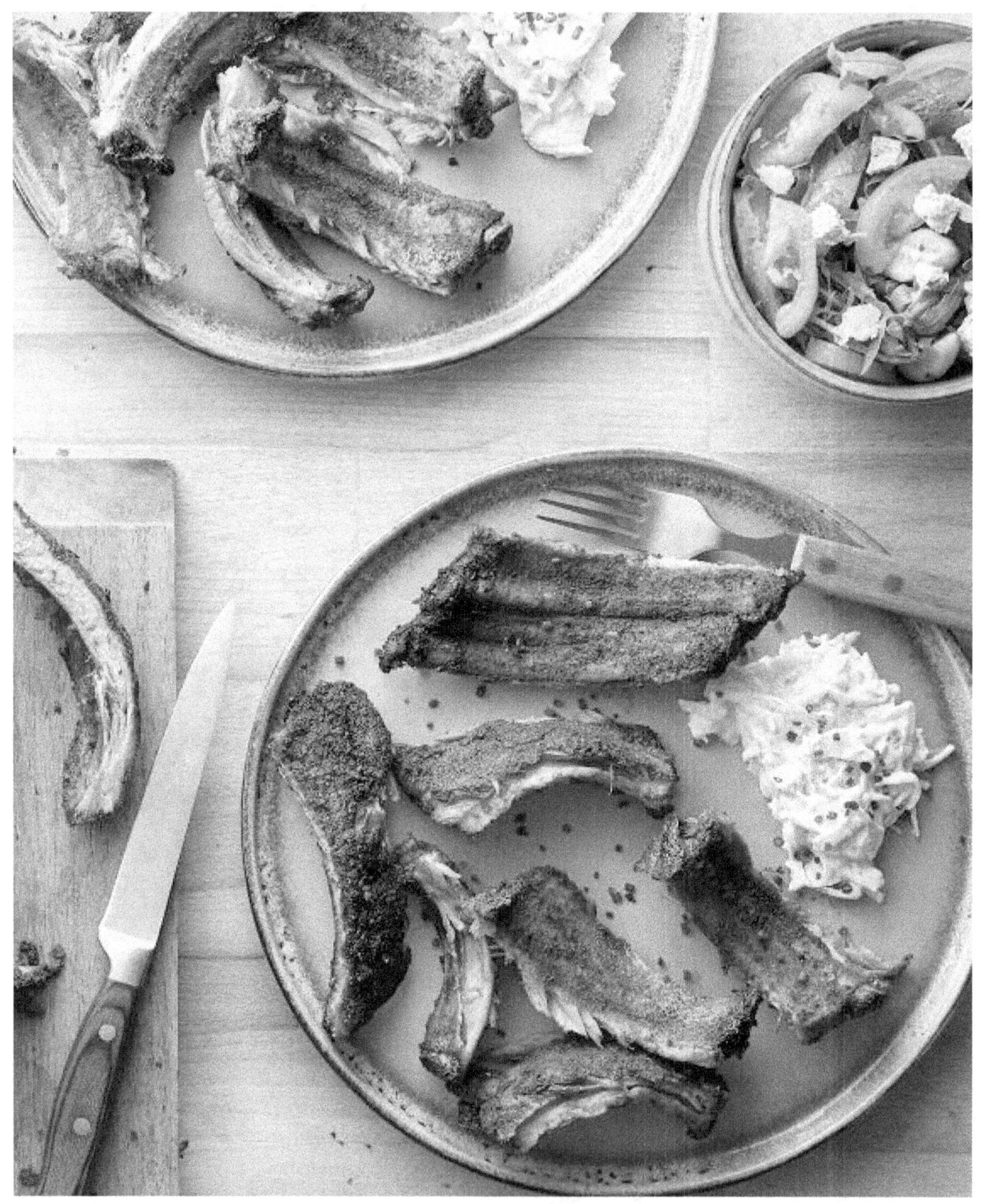

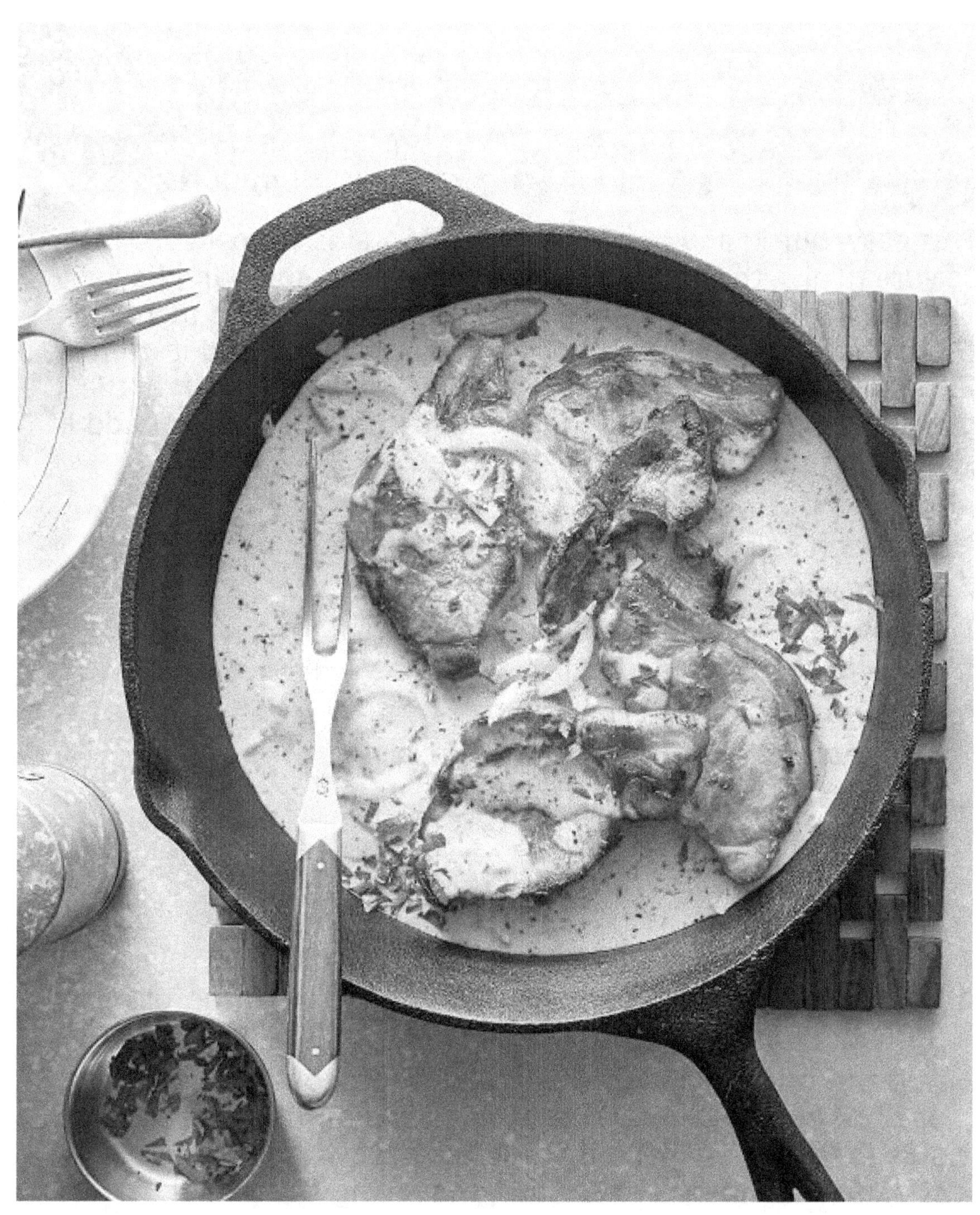

Pork Chops

This easy, quick, and delicious recipe contains almost zero carbs. Be sure to give the pork chops a good sear for color and flavor. The crushed garlic cloves are meant to be eaten with the pork chops. If desired, chop ½ of a medium onion and add in step 4 with the garlic. Cook, stirring often, for 3 minutes or until the garlic has lightly browned and the onion has softened, or add in sliced white onion in step 4, if desired.

4 bone-in pork chops

1 teaspoon salt

½ teaspoon freshly ground black pepper

1 tablespoon extra-vigin olive oil

1 tablespoon unsalted butter

8 large garlic cloves, crushed

½ cup reduced-sodium chicken broth

½ cup heavy (whipping) cream

1 teaspoon fresh lemon juice

1 tablespoon chopped fresh parsley (optional)

1. Season the pork chops with the salt and pepper.

2. In a large skillet over medium-high heat, heat the olive oil until it shimmers.

3. Add the pork chops to the skillet and cook for 3 minutes, or until browned. Flip the pork chops and sear the other side for another 3 minutes, or until browned. Transfer the cooked pork chops to a plate, reserving the skillet.

4. Add the butter to the skillet and heat until bubbly. Reduce the heat to medium and add the garlic cloves to the skillet. Cook, stirring often, for 3 minutes, or until the garlic has lightly browned.

5. Add the chicken broth, heavy cream, and lemon juice to the skillet, and heat until the mixture just comes to a boil. Reduce the heat and simmer for 2 minutes, until the sauce begins to thicken.

6. Return the pork chops to the skillet, and cook for another 5 minutes, until the sauce has thickened and the pork chops have reached an internal temperature of 145°F. Garnish the cooked pork chops with fresh parsley (if using).

PER SERVING: Calories: 333; Total fat: 25g; Total carbs: 3g; Fiber: 0g; Net carbs: 3g; Protein: 23g

Beef and Broccoli Stir-Fry

SERVES: 4 | Dairy-Free

PREP TIME: 10 minutes, plus 30 minutes to marinate | COOK TIME: 10 minutes

Slicing the meat for this stir-fry while it is still slightly frozen allows you to cut it thinly with ease. I like to use beef tenderloin for this dish, but tender cuts of beef such as sirloin, top loin, and flat iron work well, too.

1½ teaspoons sugar-free sweet chili sauce

¼ cup coconut aminos

¼ cup apple cider vinegar

1 teaspoon toasted sesame oil

1 teaspoon ginger paste

2 garlic cloves, minced

1 pound beef tenderloin, thinly sliced

2 tablespoons extra-virgin olive oil

2 cups broccoli florets

½ medium red bell pepper, seeded and cut into ¼-by-2-inch strips

½ yellow onion, thinly sliced

1 scallion, green and white parts, sliced (optional)

1. In a small bowl, combine the sweet chili sauce, coconut aminos, vinegar, sesame oil, ginger, and garlic. Reserve ¼ cup of the sauce for stir-frying.

2. Place the steak in a large resealable bag. Pour the remaining sauce over the steak. Seal and refrigerate for at least 30 minutes or up to one day.

3. In a large nonstick skillet over high heat, heat the olive oil until it shimmers. Add the beef and stir-fry for 3 minutes or until the beef has just browned. Transfer the beef to a plate and set aside, reserving the skillet.

4. To the reserved skillet, add the broccoli, bell pepper, and onion. Stir-fry for 4 minutes or until the vegetables brighten and are crisp-tender when pierced with a fork.

5. Return the beef to the pan along with the ¼ cup of reserved sauce. Toss to coat. Remove the pan from the heat. Serve, garnished with scallion (if using).

INGREDIENT TIP: If you can't find a sugar-free sweet chili sauce you like (I prefer G. Hughes Sweet Chili Sauce), substitute 1½ teaspoons (or to taste) of sriracha sauce with 1½ teaspoons of powdered natural sweetener.

PER SERVING: Calories: 390; Total fat: 30g; Total carbs: 9g; Fiber: 2g; Net carbs: 7g; Protein: 21g

Beef Burrito Bowl

Packed with protein and flavor, this burrito bowl can be served topped with a drizzle of Chipotle Ranch Dressing to boost the flavors. This recipe can easily be halved to serve just 2 people. It's a great way to use up any leftover Cauliflower Fried Rice you may have on hand.

1 pound 80/20 ground beef, crumbled

1½ teaspoons chili powder

1 teaspoon ground cumin

1 teaspoon smoked paprika

1 teaspoon salt

½ teaspoon cayenne pepper

4 cups Cauliflower Fried Rice

1 cup diced tomatoes

1 cup diced English cucumber

1 avocado, peeled, pitted, and diced

½ cup shredded full-fat cheddar cheese

½ cup chopped fresh cilantro leaves

4 tablespoons full-fat sour cream (optional)

4 tablespoons keto-friendly salsa (optional)

1. Heat a large skillet over medium-high heat. Add the ground beef and cook, stirring occasionally, for 5 minutes until it starts to brown.

2. Season the beef with the chili powder, cumin, paprika, salt, and cayenne pepper. Cook, stirring, for 5 minutes, until the beef has browned and is cooked through.

3. Divide the cauliflower rice among four serving bowls. Top each bowl with one-quarter of the beef mixture. Add ¼ cup of the tomatoes and cucumber to each bowl, and sprinkle with one-quarter of the diced avocado, 2 tablespoons of the cheddar cheese, and one-quarter of the cilantro. Serve with sour cream (if using) and salsa (if using).

VARIATION: Make this vegetarian by substituting an 8-ounce package of beef-less ground beef (I prefer Trader Joe's brand) or frozen plant-based crumbles.

PER SERVING: Calories: 440; Total fat: 30g; Total carbs: 15g; Fiber: 6g; Net carbs: 9g; Protein: 27g

Beef Tips with Creamy Mushroom Sauce

SERVES: 4 | 30 Minutes or Less, Quick Prep
PREP TIME: 10 minutes | COOK TIME: 20 minutes

These beef tips are delicious served atop a bowl Cauliflower Fried Rice or a bowl of mashed cauliflower.

1 tablespoon extra-virgin olive oil

2 pounds beef sirloin, cut into cubes

1 teaspoon salt

½ teaspoon freshly ground black pepper

1 tablespoon unsalted butter

3 large garlic cloves, sliced

8 ounces button mushrooms, sliced

16 ounces reduced-sodium beef broth

½ cup heavy (whipping) cream

1. In a large skillet over medium heat, heat the olive oil until it shimmers. Add the beef, and season with the salt and pepper. Cook, stirring occasionally, for 6 minutes, until the beef is almost cooked through.

2. Meanwhile, in another large skillet over medium heat, melt the butter. Add the garlic and cook, stirring constantly, for 1 minute, until fragrant and lightly browned.

3. Add the mushrooms to the garlic butter mixture, and then increase the heat to medium-high. Cook the mushrooms, stirring occasionally, for 7 minutes, until softened.

4. To the mushrooms, add the beef broth and the beef, and stir to combine. Bring the mixture to a simmer and cook, stirring occasionally, for 3 minutes.

5. Stir in the heavy cream. Bring the mixture to a boil, and
   cook for 1 minute or until the sauce has thickened slightly
   and is creamy.

PER SERVING: Calories: 475; Total fat: 27g; Total carbs: 4g;
Fiber: 0.5g; Net carbs: 3.5g; Protein: 55g

Sweet and Sour Meatloaf

In this meatloaf, I like to use half pork and half ground beef for the best flavor. Fat will pool around the meatloaf as it bakes. Let the meatloaf cool for 15 minutes, then gently drain the fat from the meatloaf before serving. If you don't allow the meatloaf to cool before draining the fat, the fat could cause the topping to slide right off.

Olive oil cooking spray

½ pound 80/20 ground beef

½ pound ground pork

1 cup shredded full-fat Colby jack cheese

¼ cup diced dill pickles

2 tablespoons pickle juice

¼ cup diced yellow onion

1 large egg

1 cup almond meal

¾ cup sugar-free ketchup (I use G. Hughes or Heinz)

¼ cup brown sugar natural sweetener (golden monkfruit)

2 tablespoons apple cider vinegar

2 teaspoons yellow mustard

1. Preheat the oven to 350°F. Coat a standard loaf pan with cooking spray and set aside.

2. In a large bowl, combine the beef, pork, cheese, dill pickles, pickle juice, onion, egg, and almond meal. Using your hands, mix the ingredients until just combined.

3. Transfer the meatloaf mixture to the prepared loaf, packing it evenly into the pan. Set aside.

4. In a small bowl, whisk together the ketchup, natural sweetener, vinegar, and mustard. Spread the sweet and sour sauce evenly over the meatloaf.

5. Bake the meatloaf for 50 minutes or until the internal temperature reaches 160°F. Remove the meatloaf from the oven and let cool for 15 minutes before serving.

VARIATION: If you aren't a fan of pickles, go ahead and substitute diced red or green bell pepper, and replace the pickle juice with apple cider vinegar.

PER SERVING: Calories: 356; Total fat: 26g; Total carbs 16g; Fiber: 3g; Net carbs: 5g; Protein 22g

Keto Shepherd's Pie

SERVES: **6** | Worth the Wait
PREP TIME: **15 minutes** | COOK TIME: **30 minutes**

The easiest way to make the cauliflower mixture for this recipe is to use a steamer, either on the stovetop or in the microwave. When steamed, it should be easy to pierce with a fork. Using a blender to mash the cauliflower yields a smoother texture, but a hand masher works, too.

FOR THE BEEF MIXTURE

1 tablespoon extra-virgin olive oil

2 cups diced mushrooms

½ cup diced yellow onion

½ cup diced red bell pepper

½ cup chopped asparagus

1½ pounds 80/20 ground beef

4 ounces reduced-sodium beef broth

FOR THE CAULIFLOWER MIXTURE

1 head cauliflower, cut into florets

2 tablespoons unsalted butter

1 tablespoon keto-friendly mayonnaise or Avocado Oil Mayonnaise

½ cup shredded full-fat cheddar cheese

¾ teaspoon salt

½ teaspoon freshly ground black pepper

1 teaspoon smoked paprika

TO MAKE THE BEEF MIXTURE

1. Preheat the oven to 350°F. Set aside a 9-by-13-inch baking dish.

2. In a large skillet over medium-high heat, heat the olive oil until it shimmers. Add the mushrooms, onions, bell pepper, and asparagus. Cook, stirring, for 7 minutes, until any moisture released from the mushrooms has evaporated. Transfer the vegetables to a plate and set aside, reserving the skillet.

3. Crumble the ground beef into the reserved skillet and cook, without stirring, for 5 minutes or until the beef has browned on the bottom. Then stir well, flipping the beef over to cook through. Continue to cook for 5 minutes, using a wooden spoon to break up any large clumps.

4. Add the beef broth to the cooked beef, and bring to a boil. Boil for 1 minute. Remove the skillet from the heat. Transfer the beef mixture and vegetables to the baking dish, combining and spreading evenly. Set aside.

TO MAKE THE CAULIFLOWER MIXTURE

5. Place the cauliflower in a steamer and steam for 7 minutes, until the cauliflower is fork-tender.

6. Carefully transfer the steamed cauliflower to a mixing bowl or blender. Add the butter, mayonnaise, cheese, salt, and pepper. Mix for 3 minutes or until the ingredients are fully incorporated.

7. Completely cover the beef and vegetable mixture with the cauliflower mixture, spreading evenly. Sprinkle with the paprika. Bake for 30 minutes, until the casserole is bubbling and is hot in the center.

VARIATION: Use a combination of your favorite keto-friendly vegetables in place of the asparagus or red bell pepper. Great choices would be diced radishes, chopped green beans, or chopped zucchini.

Breakfast for Dinner Burger Bowl

SERVES: **2** | 30 Minutes or Less, Quick Prep
PREP TIME: **5 minutes** | COOK TIME: **15 minutes**

This is a very big salad, made to satisfy. This salad serves two people but can be doubled to serve four with a smaller portion of beef (simply double all the ingredients, from the eggs to avocado, and portion out one-quarter of the beef mixture per serving).

1 pound 80/20 ground beef

4 slices uncured sugar-free bacon, chopped

2 tablespoons sugar-free ketchup

1 tablespoon yellow mustard

1 teaspoon salt

½ teaspoon freshly ground black pepper

1 tablespoon unsalted butter

2 large eggs

4 cups packed chopped romaine lettuce

6 cherry tomatoes, halved

1 avocado, peeled, pitted, and diced (optional)

1. Heat a large skillet over medium-high heat. Add the ground beef and bacon and cook, using a wooden spoon to occasionally break up and stir the meat mixture, for 10 minutes, until the beef has browned, and the bacon has crisped.

2. Add the ketchup, mustard, salt, and pepper to the beef mixture and stir well. Remove the pan from the heat, and set aside.

3. In a small skillet over medium heat, melt the butter. Crack the eggs into the skillet and cook for 2 minutes or until the

tops of the whites are set but the yolk is still runny.

4. Meanwhile, divide the lettuce, tomatoes, and avocado (if using) between two serving bowls and top with half of the meat mixture. Place 1 fried egg on top of each serving.

VARIATION: Serve the burger mixture over 1 cup of the Cauliflower Fried Rice instead of the lettuce and tomatoes. Top the burger bowl with 2 tablespoons Chipotle Ranch Dressing.

PER SERVING: Calories: 738; Total fat: 52g; Total carbs: 13g; Fiber: 7g; Net carbs: 6g; Protein: 55g

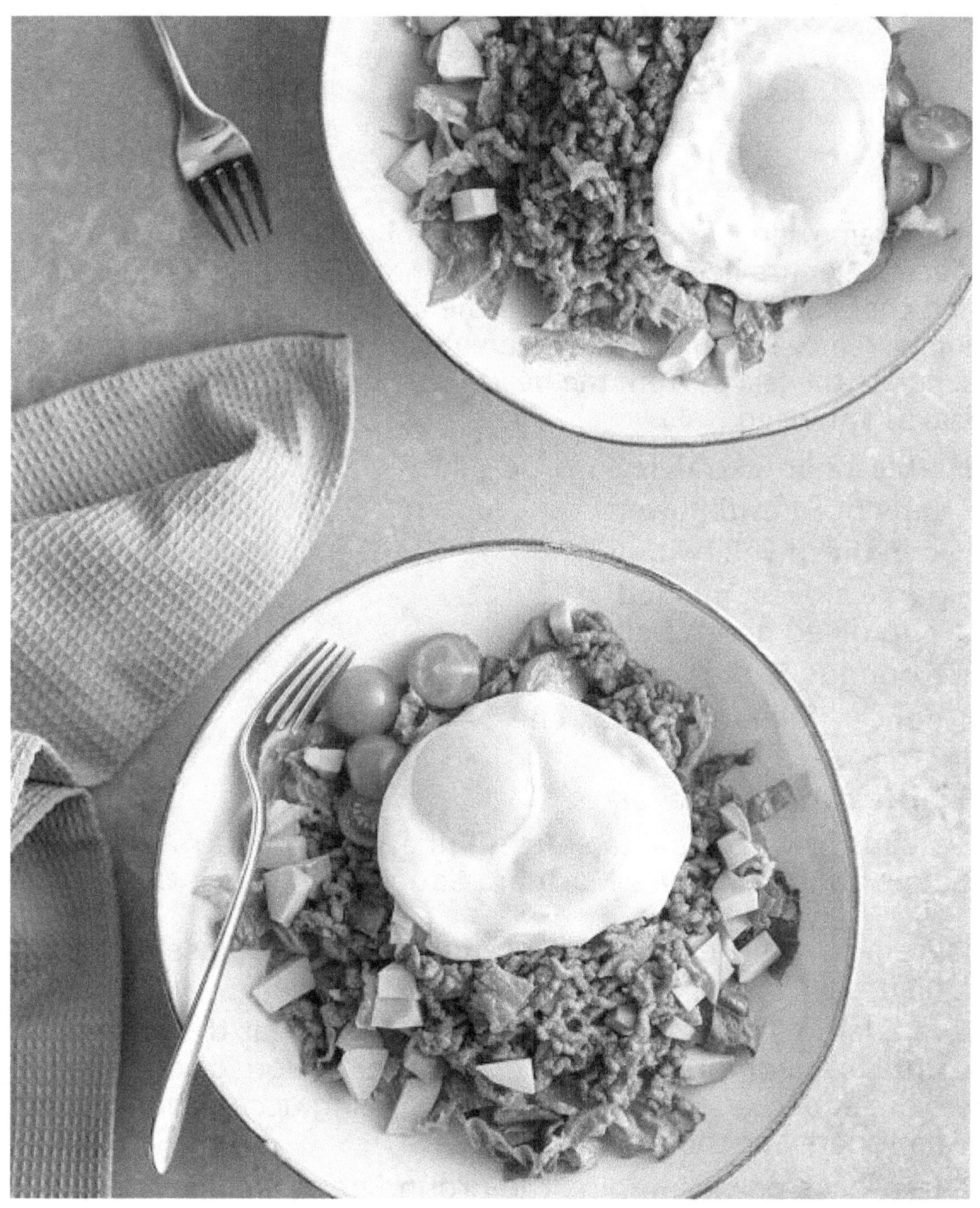

Keto Cabbage Roll Casserole

SERVES: **8** | Worth the Wait
PREP TIME: **30 minutes** | COOK TIME: **1 hour**

When removing leaves from a tight head of cabbage, it helps to place the entire head (core removed) into a pot of boiling water and cook for 2 minutes to soften the outer leaves. Then, using tongs, remove from the water, run under cool water, and carefully separate the leaves from the head. Repeat until you have the leaves you need.

1 tablespoon extra-virgin olive oil

3 cups riced cauliflower

¼ cup diced yellow onion

3 garlic cloves, minced

¼ cup diced green bell pepper

1½ pounds 80/20 ground beef

4 ounces full-fat cheddar cheese, shredded

1 large egg

8 large cabbage leaves

3½ cups low-carb pasta sauce (I like Victoria Rao's Vodka Sauce and Yo Mama's Marinara Sauce)

1. Preheat the oven to 350°F. Set aside a large glass baking dish.

2. In a large skillet over medium-high heat, heat the olive oil until it shimmers. Add the cauliflower, onion, garlic, and bell pepper. Cook for 10 minutes, stirring occasionally, until softened. Let cool for 15 minutes.

3. In a large bowl, combine the ground beef, cauliflower mixture, cheddar cheese, and egg.

4. To assemble a cabbage roll, place 1 cabbage leaf flat on your work space (if the cabbage rib is large, you may need to cut it out with a paring knife to facilitate rolling). Place about ⅓ cup of the meat mixture in the center of the cabbage leaf. Starting from the bottom edge of the cabbage leaf, roll the cabbage up and over the meat mixture. Then fold in each side of the leaf, and continue rolling to enclose the meat. Place the cabbage roll seam-side down in the baking dish. Repeat with the remaining cabbage leaves and meat mixture.

5. Pour the pasta sauce evenly over the cabbage rolls. Bake for 1 hour.

PER SERVING: Calories: 337; Total Fat: 26g; Total carbs 9g; Fiber: 2g; Net carbs: 7g; Protein 21g

Ginger Garlic Pork Meatballs

SERVES: **4** | 30 Minutes or Less, Dairy-Free
PREP TIME: **15 minutes** | COOK TIME: **15 minutes**

Enjoy these meatballs as a main meal served over Cauliflower Fried Rice or serve them as an easy appetizer for game day, holiday gatherings, and New Year's Eve parties. Just place the cooked meatballs in a slow cooker, set on warm, and enjoy the extra time you have to mingle with guests.

1½ pounds ground pork

½ cup almond meal

1 large egg

4 garlic cloves, minced

3 teaspoons sesame oil, divided

¼ cup sliced scallions, white and green parts, divided

1 tablespoon extra-virgin olive oil

1 teaspoon ginger paste

¾ cup reduced-sodium chicken broth

½ cup coconut aminos

½ cup brown sugar natural sweetener

¼ cup thinly sliced carrot

¼ teaspoon red pepper flakes (optional)

1 teaspoon toasted sesame seeds (optional)

1. In a large bowl, using your hands, combine the ground pork, almond meal, egg, garlic, 1 teaspoon of the sesame oil, and ⅛ cup of the scallions until just combined.

2. Shape the pork mixture into 1-inch meatballs (approximately 1 tablespoon).

166

3. In a large skillet over medium-high heat, heat the olive oil until it shimmers. Add the meatballs to the skillet, and cook for 3 minutes on each side, or until well browned and cooked through. Transfer the meatballs to a plate and set aside.

4. Add the remaining 2 teaspoons of sesame oil to the skillet. Swirl to coat the bottom of the pan. Add the ginger and cook, stirring constantly, for 1 minute. Stir in the chicken broth, coconut aminos, and natural sweetener. Bring the liquid to a boil, stirring constantly.

5. Return the meatballs to the skillet and toss to coat. Add the carrot and red pepper flakes (if using). Simmer for 2 minutes or until the sauce has reduced and thickened. Sprinkle with sesame seeds (if using).

PER SERVING: Calories: 487; Total fat: 38g; Total carbs: 22g; Fiber: 2g; Net carbs: 8g; Protein 38g

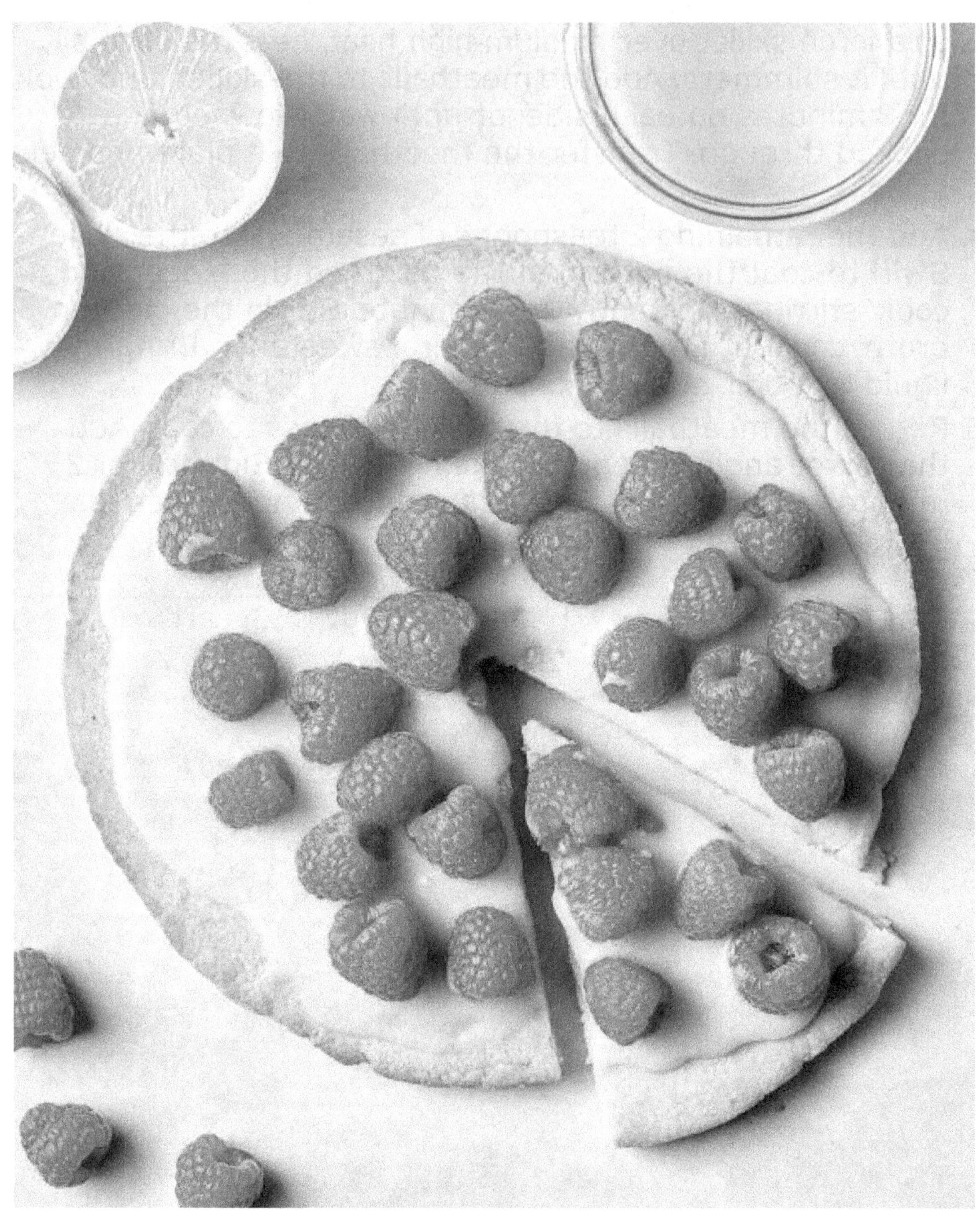

Raspberry Lemon Fruit Pizza

&

<u>Desserts</u>

<u>Tiramisu</u>
<u>Rhubarb Dream Bars</u>
<u>Quick Strawberry Shortcake</u>
<u>Chocolate Mayonnaise Cake</u>
<u>Raspberry Lemon Fruit Pizza</u>
<u>Spiced Mug Cake</u>
<u>Chocolate Bark with Walnuts</u>
<u>Chewy Chocolate Chip Cookies</u>

Tiramisu

This scaled-down version of tiramisu fits the keto diet and is delicious! When cooking the cake layer in the microwave, use a coffee mug similar in size to your serving dish. That way the cake discs will be easier to layer in your final assembly.

FOR THE CAKE LAYER

2 tablespoons instant coffee

1 tablespoon boiling water

2 tablespoons unsalted butter

½ cup powdered natural sweetener

2 tablespoons coconut flour

2 teaspoons baking powder

⅛ teaspoon salt

2 tablespoons almond flour

2 large eggs

2 teaspoons coconut oil

2 teaspoons brandy (optional)

FOR THE MASCARPONE FILLING

2 large eggs

2 teaspoons pure vanilla extract

¼ cup powdered natural sweetener

⅛ teaspoon salt

1 cup mascarpone cheese, room temperature

1 tablespoon unsweetened cocoa powder (optional)

1. In a small bowl, combine the coffee, boiling water, and butter. Stir until the coffee has dissolved and the butter has melted. Set aside.

2. In another small bowl, combine the natural sweetener, coconut flour, baking powder, salt, and almond flour. Add the coffee mixture and the eggs to the flour mixture, stirring until completely combined.

3. Grease 4 coffee mugs with the coconut oil. Divide the cake batter evenly between the 2 mugs. Place the mugs in the microwave and cook on high for 1 minute or until the cake is just dry on the top.

4. Let the cakes rest for 2 minutes. To release the cakes, invert the mugs onto a plate. Set aside to cool completely.

TO MAKE THE MASCARPONE FILLING

5. Separate the egg whites from the yolks, placing the white and yolks into two separate bowls. Using a hand mixer, whisk the egg whites for 4 minutes or until stiff peaks form.

6. To the egg yolks, add the vanilla, natural sweetener, and salt. Whisk for 2 minutes, or until pale in color and thick in texture.

7. Add the mascarpone cheese to the egg yolk mixture. Whisk until well combined.

8. Fold the egg white mixture into the cheese mixture, just until combined.

TO ASSEMBLE

9. Cut each cake in half crosswise so you end up with 8 even discs.

10. Place one-eighth of the mascarpone mixture in each of 4 serving glasses (similar in size to the coffee mugs).

11. Place 1 cake disc on top of each mascarpone layer. Drizzle ½ teaspoon brandy (if using) evenly over each cake.

12. Divide the remaining mascarpone filling evenly on top of each cake disc. Using a tea strainer or fine-mesh sieve, lightly dust the cocoa powder (if using) evenly over each tiramisu. Serve.

FLAVOR BOOST: For a nutty flavor, substitute ground hazelnut flour for the almond flour, and use hazelnut-flavored instant coffee.

PER SERVING: Calories: 415; Total fat: 39g; Total carbs: 39g; Fiber: 2g; Net carbs: 1g; Protein: 11g

RHubarb Dream Bars

Keto shortbread serves as a delicious base for a rhubarb custard filling. Covered with a cream cheese and whipped cream topping, this decadent dessert is perfect for special celebrations.

FOR THE CRUST

Olive oil cooking spray

1 cup almond flour

¼ cup coconut flour

¼ cup granulated natural sweetener

½ teaspoon salt

6 tablespoons unsalted butter, melted

FOR THE FILLING

4 large eggs

1½ cups granulated natural sweetener

½ cup heavy (whipping) cream

½ cup unsweetened almond milk

1 teaspoon pure vanilla extract

1 teaspoon xanthan gum

5 cups diced rhubarb

FOR THE TOPPING

8 ounces cream cheese, softened

½ cup powdered natural sweetener

½ teaspoon pure vanilla extract

2 cups heavy (whipping) cream, whipped

TO MAKE THE CRUST

1. Preheat the oven to 350°F. Coat a 13-by-9-inch baking dish with the cooking spray and set aside.

2. In a medium bowl, using two forks or pastry blender, combine the almond flour, coconut flour, natural sweetener, salt, and butter until the mixture resembles a coarse meal.

3. Press the flour mixture into the prepared baking dish. Bake for 15 minutes or until the crust is golden.

TO MAKE THE FILLING

4. Meanwhile, in a large bowl, using a hand mixer, whisk together the eggs, natural sweetener, heavy cream, almond milk, and vanilla.

5. Sprinkle the xanthan gum over the egg mixture. Whisk well until combined. Stir in the rhubarb.

6. Pour the egg mixture over the partially baked crust. Return the dish to the oven and bake for 50 minutes or until the custard has set and a knife inserted into the center comes out clean. Remove the pan from the oven and let cool completely.

TO MAKE THE TOPPING

7. In a medium bowl, using a hand mixer on medium speed, combine the cream cheese, natural sweetener, and vanilla until smooth.

8. Using a spatula, fold in the heavy cream. Spread the topping evenly over the completely cooled bars. Store in the refrigerator for up to 3 days.

INGREDIENT TIP: For the filling: Xanthan gum helps thicken the custard, but it can be omitted without changing the quality of the dessert (the filling won't be as firm without it). For the topping: You can omit the cream cheese from the topping for a sweetened whipped cream (here) topping.

PER SERVING: Calories: 254; Total fat: 25g; Total carbs: 29g;
Fiber: 1.5g; Net carbs: 3.5g; Protein 5g

Quick Strawberry Shortcake

A slightly sweetened biscuit topped with fresh sliced strawberries and whipped cream makes the perfect quick dessert. If you don't have buttermilk on hand, try adding 1 teaspoon of apple cider vinegar to ¼ cup almond milk. Set aside for 5 minutes, then use as you would the buttermilk.

2 cups hulled and sliced strawberries

⅛ cup powdered natural sweetener

¾ cup almond flour

¼ cup coconut flour

2 tablespoons granulated natural sweetener

¾ teaspoon baking powder

⅛ teaspoon salt

1 teaspoon cream of tartar

¼ cup buttermilk

1 large egg

2 tablespoons unsalted butter, melted

½ teaspoon pure vanilla extract

½ cup whipped cream (optional, here)

1. Preheat the oven to 350°F. Line a baking sheet with parchment paper and set aside.

2. In a small bowl, combine the strawberries and powdered natural sweetener. Set aside.

3. In a medium bowl, whisk together the almond flour, coconut flour, natural sweetener, baking powder, salt, and cream of tartar.

4. Add the buttermilk, egg, butter, and vanilla to the flour mixture, and stir until combined.

5. Drop heaping tablespoons of the dough onto the prepared baking sheet. Bake for 20 minutes or until the biscuits have browned and a toothpick inserted in the center comes out clean. Remove the sheet from the oven and let cool completely.

6. To serve, slice the biscuits in half and top each with ½ cup of the strawberries and 2 tablespoons of the whipped cream (if using).

INGREDIENT TIP: For more berry flavor, combine the berries and natural sweetener ahead of time and refrigerate for up to 12 hours before serving.

PER SERVING: Calories: 258; Total fat: 19g; Total carbs: 15g; Fiber: 6g; Net carbs: 9g; Protein: 8g

Chocolate Mayonnaise Cake

SERVES: 6 | 30 Minutes or Less, One Pot, Quick Prep
PREP TIME: 10 minutes | COOK TIME: 20 minutes

This moist and delicious chocolate mayonnaise cake is a personal favorite of mine. The mayonnaise adds a nice tang to the cake and brings out the intense flavor of the chocolate. I prefer using Hershey's Cocoa powder for this recipe.

1 teaspoon coconut oil

¾ cup almond flour

½ cup powdered natural sweetener

¼ cup plus 1 tablespoon coconut flour

⅓ cup unsweetened cocoa powder

1 tablespoon baking powder

¾ cup keto-friendly mayonnaise or Avocado Oil Mayonnaise

3 large eggs

6 tablespoons water

1½ teaspoons pure vanilla extract

1. Preheat the oven to 350°F. Coat an 8-inch cake pan with the coconut oil and set aside.
2. In a medium bowl, combine the almond flour, natural sweetener, coconut flour, cocoa powder, and baking powder.
3. Add the mayonnaise, eggs, water, and vanilla to the flour mixture. Stir well.
4. Using a spatula, scrape the cake batter into the prepared cake pan. Bake for 20 minutes or until the cake is just firm to the touch. Remove the pan from the oven and let cool completely.

 For even more decadence, serve with homemade whipped cream: In a bowl, combine 1 cup heavy cream and ¼ cup powdered natural sweetener. Using a hand mixer, whisk until the cream stabilizes and forms soft peaks. Top the cooled cake with dollops of whipped cream.

Raspberry Lemon Fruit Pizza

SERVES: 8 | Worth the Wait

PREP TIME: 15 minutes, plus 30 minutes to chill | COOK TIME: 25 minutes

The cookie base for this sweet pizza is similar to shortbread. It's just soft enough to cut but firm enough to hold in your hands. When making the lemon curd, a double boiler is preferred, but a heat-safe bowl that just fits inside a saucepan will work, too.

FOR THE COOKIE BASE

2 ounces cream cheese, room temperature

6 tablespoons unsalted butter, room temperature

½ cup granulated natural sweetener

1 teaspoon pure vanilla extract

2 cups almond flour

2 tablespoons coconut flour

½ teaspoon salt

FOR THE LEMON CURD

½ cup fresh lemon juice

1 cup powdered natural sweetener

3 large eggs

4 tablespoons unsalted butter

2 teaspoon freshly grated lemon zest

2 cups fresh raspberries (optional, for topping)

TO MAKE THE COOKIE BASE

1. Preheat the oven to 350°F. Line a large baking sheet with parchment paper and set aside.

2. In a large bowl, using a hand mixer on medium speed, cream together the cream cheese, butter, natural

sweetener, and vanilla.

3. Add the almond flour, coconut flour, and salt to the cheese mixture, and mix until completely incorporated.

4. Scrape the cookie dough onto the prepared baking sheet. Flatten with the palm of your hands, and then cover with another piece of parchment. Using a rolling pin, roll out the dough to a ½-inch-thick circle. Discard the top piece of parchment.

5. Bake for 25 minutes or until the dough is lightly browned around the edges, the center of the cookie is dry on the top, and a toothpick comes out clean when inserted into the center of the dough. Remove the pan from the oven and let the cookie cool completely.

TO MAKE THE LEMON CURD

6. While the cookie base bakes, in a double boiler over medium-high heat, whisk together the lemon juice, natural sweetener, and eggs for 2 minutes, until the egg mixture is pale yellow and the ingredients are well incorporated.

7. Stir constantly for 10 minutes, until the curd thickens.

8. Remove the pan from the heat, and stir in the butter and lemon zest. Keep stirring until the butter is melted and the mixture is creamy. Cover (see Tip) and refrigerate for at least 30 minutes, or until ready to use.

TO ASSEMBLE

9. Spread 1 cup of the lemon curd evenly over the cooled cookie crust.

10. Sprinkle raspberries evenly over the lemon curd. Store any unused curd in an airtight container in the refrigerator for up to one week.

INGREDIENT TIP: To prevent a skin from forming on top of the lemon curd while cooling, pour the curd into a small bowl and then place a piece of plastic wrap directly on the surface of the curd.

Spiced Mug Cake

My favorite way to serve this mug cake is with a tablespoon of sugar-free whipped cream or keto-friendly vanilla ice cream. I also like to cut the cooled mug cake in half crosswise and spread a tablespoon of Chia Seed Jam in the center, then top with a tablespoon of whipped cream (here) and sprinkle with more cinnamon to garnish.

1 tablespoon unsalted butter

¼ cup almond flour

2 tablespoons brown sugar natural sweetener

½ teaspoon baking powder

¼ teaspoon ground cinnamon, plus more for garnish

⅛ teaspoon ground ginger

⅛ teaspoon ground nutmeg

Pinch ground cloves

Pinch salt

1 large egg

½ teaspoon pure vanilla extract

1. Melt the butter in a microwave-safe mug for 10 seconds. To the mug, add the almond flour, natural sweetener, baking powder, cinnamon, ginger, nutmeg, cloves, salt, egg, and vanilla. Mix until smooth.
2. Microwave on high for 1 minute, until the cake is just firm. Let cool slightly before serving.

PER SERVING: Calories: 314; Total fat: 28g; Total carbs: 4.5g; Fiber: 3g; Net carbs: 1.5g; Protein: 11g

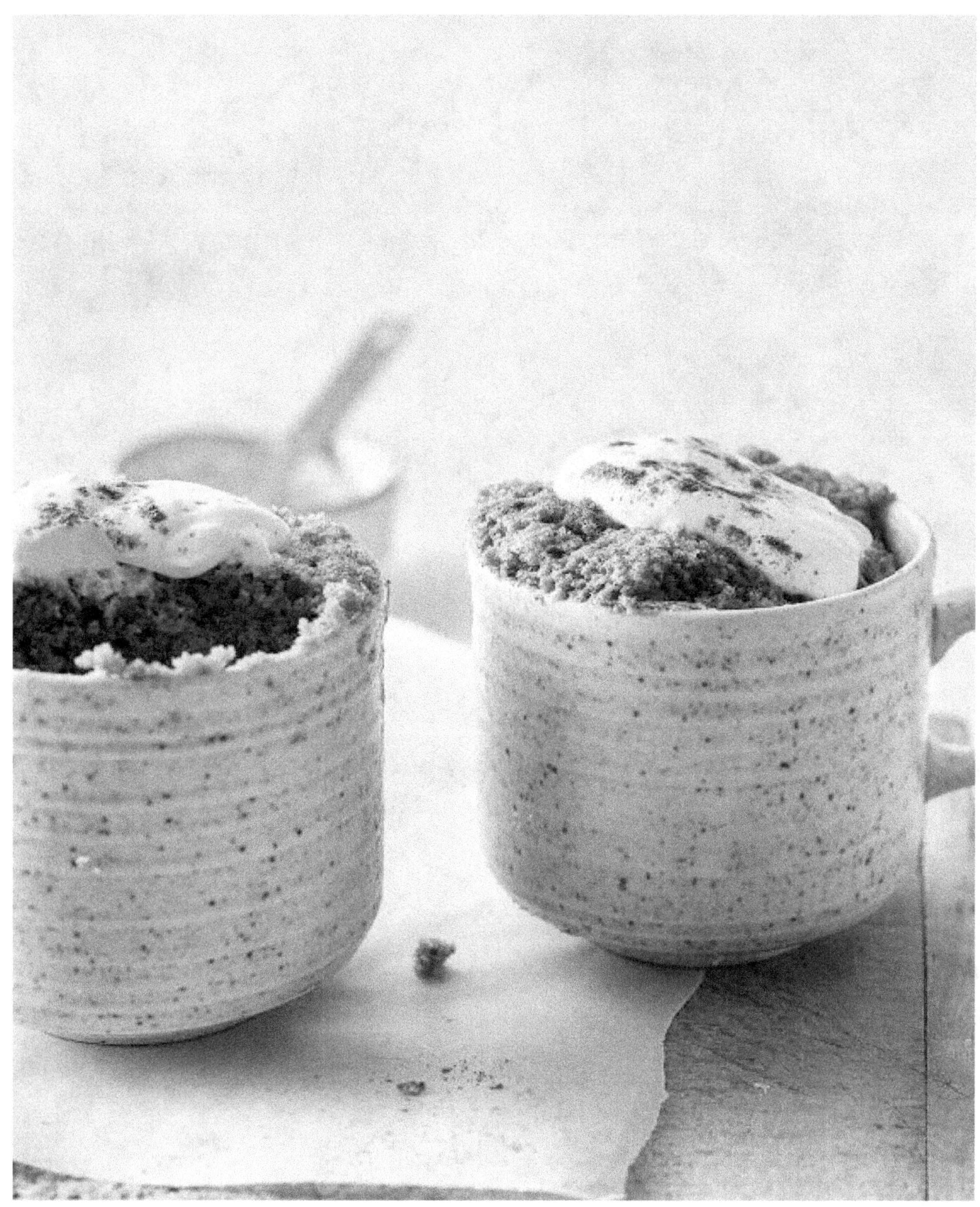

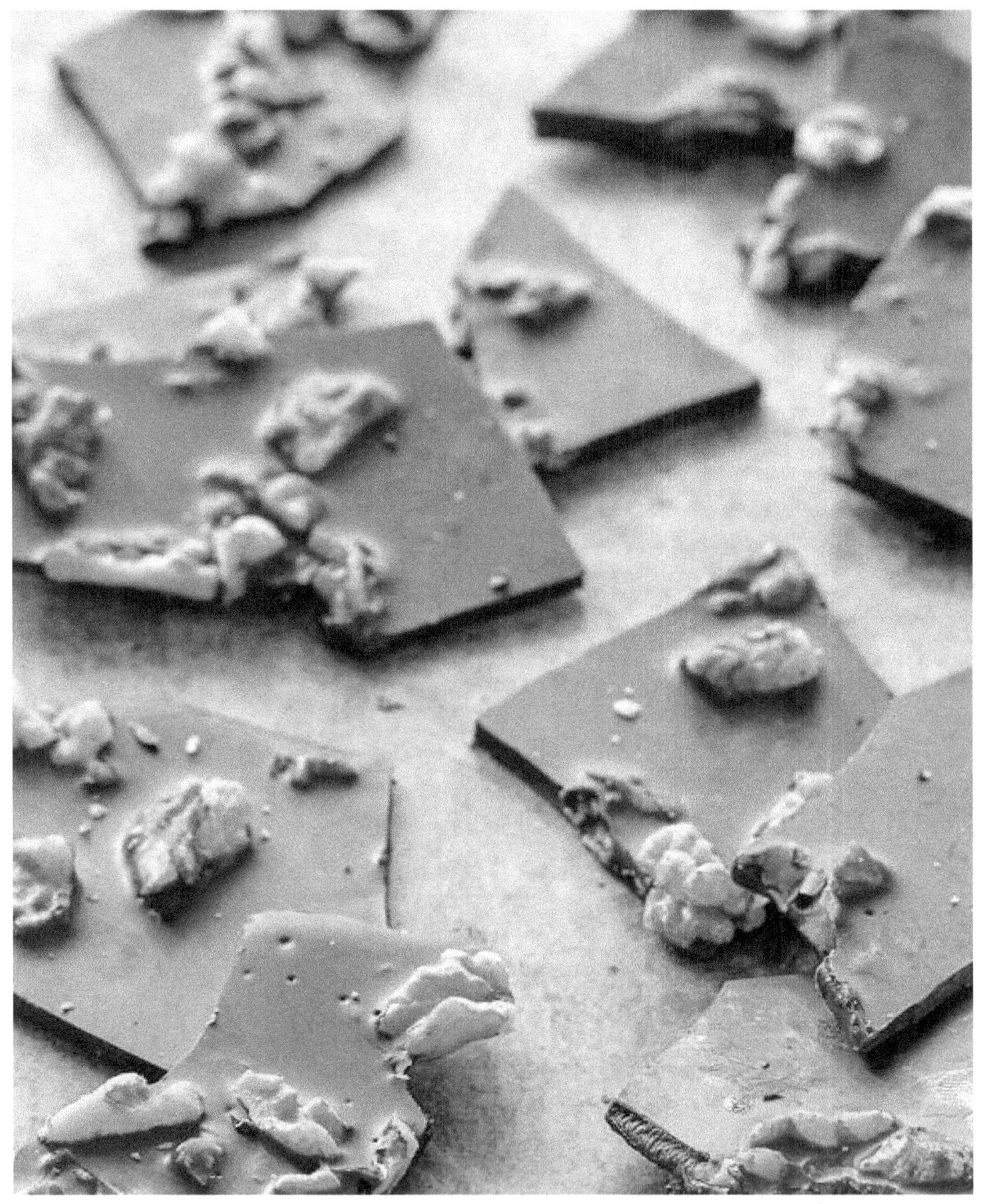

CHocolate Bark witH Walnuts

SERVES: 8 | 5 Ingredients or Less, 30 Minutes or Less, Dairy-Free, Quick Prep, Vegetarian
PREP TIME: 5 minutes | COOK TIME: 5 minutes

I always melt the chocolate for this recipe in a double boiler. If you don't own one, use a glass bowl that just fits over a saucepan. The steam from the water will melt the chocolate evenly and smoothly. I don't recommend using the microwave because the chocolate could burn and the result will taste bitter.

2 cups sugar-free dark chocolate chips

1 cup walnut halves, chopped

1. Line a large baking sheet with parchment paper. Set aside.

2. Fill a saucepan with 1 to 2 inches of water. Place a double boiler or shallow heat-safe bowl over top, making sure that the water does not touch the bottom of the bowl. Place the saucepan on the stove over medium heat.

3. Place the chocolate chips in the double boiler. As the water simmers and steams, it will melt the chocolate. Using a rubber spatula, stir the chocolate until completely melted and smooth.

4. Pour the melted chocolate onto the prepared baking sheet. Using an offset spatula or butter knife, spread the chocolate into a ¼-inch-thin layer. Immediately sprinkle the chopped walnuts evenly over the top of the melted chocolate. Set the pan aside to cool completely.

5. Once the chocolate has cooled completely, break it into pieces. Store in an airtight container for up to two weeks.

PER SERVING: Calories: 104; Total fat: 10g; Total carbs: 13g; Fiber: 6g; Net carbs: 4g; Protein: 2g

Chewy Chocolate Chip Cookies

MAKES: 12 cookies | 30 Minutes or Less, Quick Prep
PREP TIME: 10 minutes | COOK TIME: **15 minutes**

These cookies are fragile when hot, so it is important to let them cool completely before removing them from the baking sheet. Xanthan gum is a thickening agent often used in keto cooking for making gravies. I discovered that it also adds a little chew to cookies!

1½ cups almond flour

½ cup brown sugar natural sweetener

1 teaspoon xanthan gum

1 teaspoon baking powder

½ cup unsalted butter, melted

1 large egg

1 teaspoon pure vanilla extract

½ cup sugar-free chocolate chips

1. Preheat the oven to 350°F. Line a large baking sheet with parchment paper.

2. In a medium bowl, whisk together the almond flour, natural sweetener, xanthan gum, and baking powder. Set aside.

3. In a small bowl, whisk together the butter, egg, and vanilla. Gradually add the wet ingredients to the dry ingredients, and mix until well combined. Using a spatula, fold in the chocolate chips.

4. Drop tablespoons of the dough onto the prepared baking sheet, spacing them at least 2 inches apart. Bake for 15 minutes or until golden brown. Remove the pan from the

oven and let the cookies cool completely on the baking sheet. The cookies will keep in an airtight container in the refrigerator for up to three months.

VARIATION: Any sugar-free flavored chip can be used in place of the chocolate chips. Also for some crunch and nutty flavor, fold ½ cup of chopped walnuts or pecans into the dough at the end of step 3.

PER SERVING (1 COOKIE): Calories: 187; Total fat: 17g; Total carbs: 4g; Fiber: 2g; Net carbs: 2g; Protein: 4g

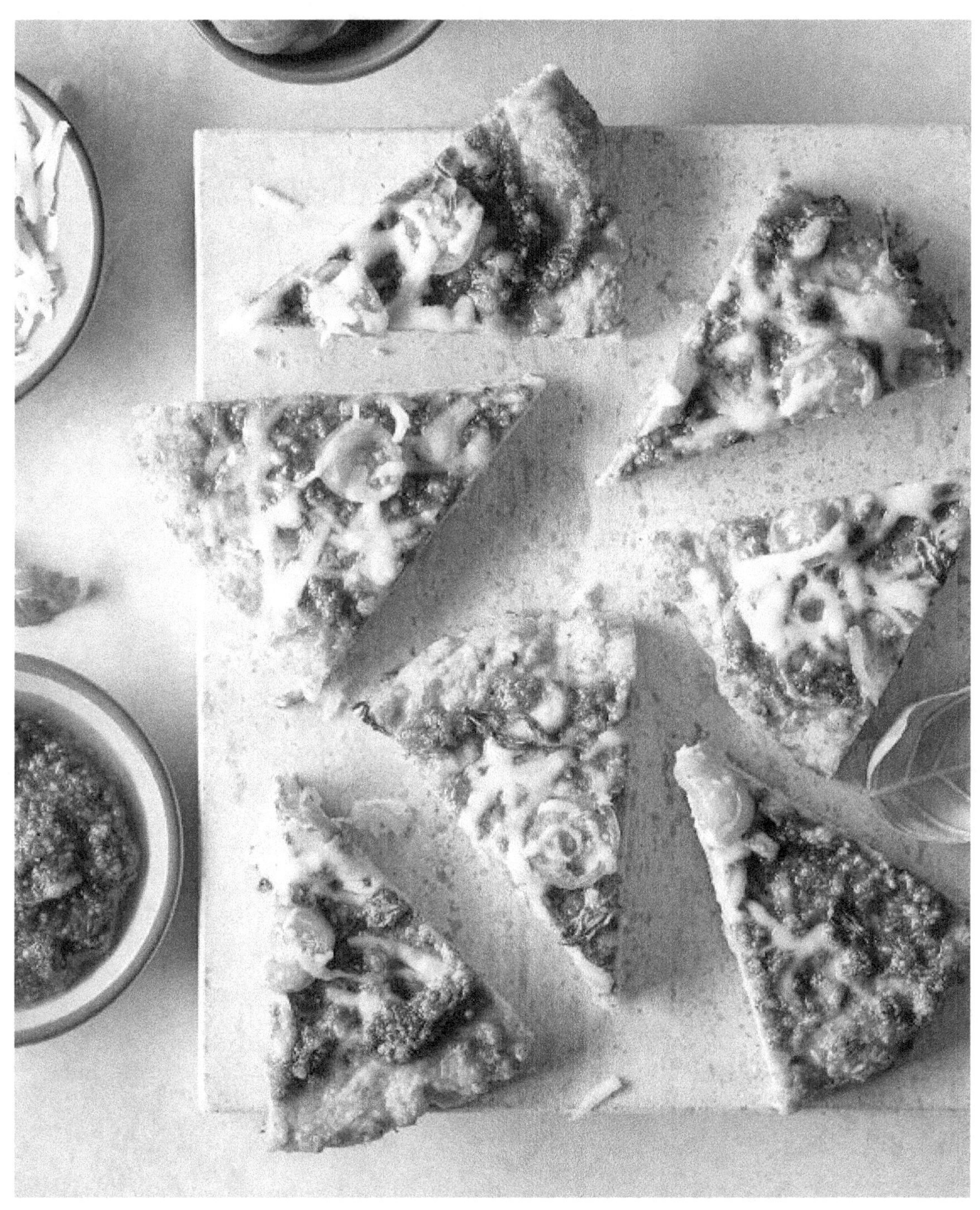

Chicken Pizza Crust

9

Sauces and Keto Staples

Avocado Oil Mayonnaise
Chipotle Ranch Dressing
Cilantro Lime Vinaigrette
Keto Maple Syrup
Fry Dipping Sauce
Chia Seed Jam
Cauliflower Tortillas
Pesto
Chicken Pizza Crust

Avocado Oil Mayonnaise

MAKES: **1 cup** | 5 Ingredients or Less, 30 Minutes or Less, Dairy-Free, One Pot, Quick Prep, Vegetarian
PREP TIME: **5 minutes**

Raw eggs are nutrient-dense and packed with protein, fat, vitamins, and minerals, with the yolk containing most of the nutrients. Using pasteurized eggs lessens the possibility of salmonella. The yolk used in this recipe lends a creamy, buttery flavor, and the smoked paprika adds a little depth to the mayonnaise.

1 large egg yolk

1½ tablespoons fresh lemon juice

1 teaspoon Dijon mustard

½ teaspoon salt

½ teaspoon smoked paprika

¾ cup avocado oil

1. In a medium bowl, whisk together the egg yolk, lemon juice, mustard, salt, and paprika until frothy.
2. While whisking, gradually drizzle the oil, about 1 tablespoon at a time, into the egg mixture, whisking constantly, until the mayonnaise is thick and the oil is fully incorporated.
3. Refrigerate in an airtight container for up to one week.

FLAVOR BOOST: For a different flavor profile, substitute an equal amount of fresh lime juice or apple cider vinegar for the lemon juice.

Chipotle Ranch Dressing

This dressing is very versatile and ready in just 10 minutes. Chilling the dressing in the refrigerator for at least 30 minutes before serving allows the flavors to meld. If you are unsure about the taste of chipotle, start with just 1 pepper and 1 tablespoon of the adobo sauce and adjust accordingly.

1 cup keto-friendly mayonnaise or <u>Avocado Oil Mayonnaise</u>

2 canned chipotle peppers, finely chopped

2 tablespoons adobo sauce

2 garlic cloves, minced

2 teaspoons powdered natural sweetener

1 tablespoon fresh lime juice

1 teaspoon smoked paprika

1. In a medium bowl, combine the mayonnaise, chipotle peppers, adobo sauce, garlic, natural sweetener, lime juice, and paprika. Stir well.
2. Refrigerate in an airtight container for up to two weeks.

INGREDIENT TIP: You can substitute ½ cup of full-fat Greek yogurt or sour cream for the mayonnaise.

PER SERVING (1 TABLESPOON): Calories: 83; Total fat: 9g; Total carbs: 0.5g; Fiber: 0g; Net carbs: 0.5g; Protein: 0g

Cilantro Lime Vinaigrette

MAKES: ½ cup | 5 Ingredients or Less, 30 Minutes or Less, Dairy-Free, One Pot, Quick Prep, Vegetarian
PREP TIME: **5 minutes**

This is one of my favorite dressings to enjoy on a garden salad. It is also an excellent marinade for grilled shrimp and a lovely dressing for Seared Scallops. Shaking this up in a jar works really well, but if you prefer the cilantro to be more finely incorporated, place all the ingredients in a blender and blend until smooth.

¼ cup lime juice

¼ cup extra-virgin olive oil

2 garlic cloves, minced

1 teaspoon powdered natural sweetener

½ teaspoon salt

½ teaspoon ground cumin

2 tablespoons chopped fresh cilantro leaves

1. In a pint-size jar with a lid, combine the lime juice, olive oil, garlic, natural sweetener, salt, cumin, and cilantro. Cover and shake well.

2. Refrigerate for up to one week.

VARIATION: An equal amount of fresh lemon juice or apple cider vinegar can be substituted for the lime juice.

PER SERVING (1 TABLESPOON): Calories: 63; Total fat: 6.5g; Total carbs: 1g; Fiber: 0g; Net carbs: 1g; Protein: 0g

Keto Maple Syrup

MAKES: **2½ cups** | 5 Ingredients or Less, 30 Minutes or Less, One Pot, Quick Prep, Vegetarian
PREP TIME: **5 minutes** | COOK TIME: **5 minutes**

Pure maple syrup is high in calories and carbs so you should avoid it on keto. Thankfully, this syrup is a delicious alternative. Drizzle over Chocolate Chip Chaffles and use instead of icing on Cinnamon Roll Pancakes. Xanthan gum works to thicken the syrup. For best results, lightly sprinkle the xanthan gum over the syrup while whisking constantly to avoid clumps of gum.

¾ cup brown sugar natural sweetener

¼ cup powdered natural sweetener

2¼ cups water

1 tablespoon unsalted butter

1 teaspoon imitation maple extract

¼ teaspoon salt

1 teaspoon xanthan gum

1. In a large saucepan over medium-high heat, combine the brown sugar natural sweetener, powdered sugar natural sweetener, and water. Stir well. Bring the mixture to a boil while stirring occasionally. Once boiling, reduce the heat to low.

2. Add the butter, maple extract, and salt to the sugar mixture. Whisk until combined.

3. While whisking, sprinkle the xanthan gum over the syrup mixture. Whisk until the gum is fully incorporated. Increase the heat to medium, and continue to cook for 2 minutes, until the syrup has thickened.

4. Remove the syrup from the heat and cool completely. Store in an airtight container in the refrigerator up to two weeks.

VARIATION: Make cinnamon maple syrup: Add 1 teaspoon of cinnamon with the brown sugar in step 1.

PER SERVING (2 TABLESPOONS): Calories: 6.5; Total fat: 0.5g; Total carbs: 0.5g; Fiber: 0g; Net carbs: 0.5g; Protein: 0g

Fry Dipping Sauce

MAKES: **1 cup** | 5 Ingredients or Less, 30 Minutes or Less,
Dairy-Free, One Pot, Quick Prep, Vegetarian
PREP TIME: **5 minutes**

The tangy sweet-and-savory flavor of this dipping sauce is hard to resist. It's a great topping for burgers, and my entire family loves to dip the Zucchini Fries, Onion Rings, and Keto Chicken Nuggets in it! You can also use this in place of the mayonnaise dressing in the Sweet and Spicy Broccoli Salad.

½ cup keto-friendly mayonnaise or Avocado Oil Mayonnaise

¼ cup sugar-free ketchup

3 tablespoons powdered natural sweetener

2 teaspoons yellow mustard

2 teaspoons Dijon mustard

¼ cup fresh lime juice

½ teaspoon cayenne pepper

1. In a small bowl, whisk together the mayonnaise, ketchup, natural sweetener, yellow mustard, Dijon mustard, lime juice, and cayenne pepper, until the natural sweetener has fully dissolved.

2. Transfer the sauce to an airtight container and refrigerate until ready to serve, or up to one week.

VARIATION: For a slightly different flavor, substitute lemon juice for the lime juice, and chili powder for the cayenne pepper.

PER SERVING (1 TABLESPOON): Calories: 51; Total fat: 5g; Total carbs: 1.5g; Fiber: 0g; Net carbs: 1.5g; Protein: g

Chia Seed Jam

Chia seeds are an excellent thickening agent, and the best thing is how good they are for you: They are full of nutrition and packed with fiber, protein, and omega-3 fatty acids. Enjoy this jam slathered over keto-friendly breads, or use in place of the lemon curd and raspberries in Raspberry Lemon Fruit Pizza.

3 cups fresh raspberries, blackberries, or sliced hulled
 strawberries

¼ cup powdered natural sweetener

2 tablespoons water

2 tablespoons chia seeds

1 tablespoon fresh lemon juice

¼ teaspoon pure vanilla extract

⅛ teaspoon pure orange extract (optional)

1. In a medium saucepan over medium-high heat, combine the berries, natural sweetener, and water. Cook, mashing the berries with a potato masher or fork, until the berries have fully broken down.

2. Add the chia seeds to the pan, and cook for 5 minutes or until the jam begins to thicken.

3. Remove the pan from the heat. Stir in the lemon juice, vanilla, and orange extract (if using). Set aside to cool completely.

4. Transfer the jam to an airtight jar and refrigerate for up to 2 weeks.

INGREDIENT TIP: **If you prefer your jam without seeds, press the berry mixture through a fine-mesh sieve (using the back of a spoon) before adding the chia seeds in step 2.**

PER SERVING (1 TABLESPOON): Calories: 18.5; Total fat: 0.5g; Total carbs: 3.5g; Fiber: 2g; Net carbs: 1.5g; Protein: 0g

Cauliflower Tortillas

MAKES: **6 tortillas** | 5 Ingredients or Less, 30 Minutes or Less, Dairy-Free, Quick Prep, Vegetarian
PREP TIME: **5 minutes** | COOK TIME: **15 minutes**

Traditional corn and flour tortillas are not keto-friendly (they contain too many carbs), but these cauliflower tortillas work like a charm and are tasty, too. For best results when serving, brown the cauliflower tortillas before using them: Placing a baked tortilla in a hot skillet over medium-high heat. Cook for 1 minute on each side, until warmed. Enjoy with your favorite fillings.

2 large eggs

2 cups riced cauliflower, steamed, and squeezed dry (see Tip)

2 tablespoons chopped fresh parsley leaves

½ teaspoon freshly grated lemon zest

1 tablespoon fresh lemon juice

½ teaspoon salt

¼ teaspoon freshly ground black pepper

1. Preheat the oven to 375°F. Line a large baking sheet with parchment paper and set aside.

2. In a medium bowl, whisk the eggs until foamy. Add the cauliflower, parsley, lemon zest, lemon juice, salt, and pepper. Mix until well combined.

3. Scoop ⅓ cup of the cauliflower mixture and, using your hands, flatten and shape it into a small tortilla-like round. Place on top of the parchment-lined baking sheet. Repeat with the remaining cauliflower mixture (you should end up with 6 tortillas).

4. Bake for 10 minutes. Remove the pan from the oven and carefully flip each tortilla.

5. Return the pan to the oven, and cook the tortillas for an additional 7 minutes, or until the tortillas have completely set and are lightly browned.

6. Remove the pan from the oven and let the tortillas cool completely on the baking sheet.

7. Store any leftover tortillas in the refrigerator, covered, for up to 3 days.

COOKING TIP: It's important to squeeze out as much of the liquid from the steamed riced cauliflower as possible. To steam, place the riced cauliflower in a microwave-safe bowl and cook on high for 6 minutes, stirring halfway through. Carefully transfer the steamed cauliflower to the center of a clean dish towel, fold up the sides, and twist and wring out as much liquid as possible. I recommend wearing gloves when doing this to prevent steam burns.

PER SERVING (1 TORTILLA): Calories: 33.5; Total fat: 1.5g; Total carbs: 2g; Fiber: 1g; Net carbs: 1g; Protein: 3g

Pesto

MAKES: **2 cups** | 5 Ingredients or Less, 30 Minutes or Less, One Pot, Quick Prep, Vegetarian
PREP TIME: **15 minutes**

Pesto is naturally keto-friendly! When making pesto, be sure to scrape down the sides of the bowl several times during processing to ensure all the ingredients are fully incorporated. Pesto makes an excellent topping for Chicken Pizza Crust and Egg in a Hole Pepper Rings.

2 cups fresh basil leaves

½ cup pine nuts

¾ cup freshly grated Parmesan cheese

3 large garlic cloves

½ teaspoon salt

¼ teaspoon freshly ground black pepper

½ cup extra-vigin olive oil

1. Place the basil in a food processor or blender, and pulse several times until finely chopped.

2. Add the pine nuts, Parmesan, garlic, salt, and pepper. Pulse several more times, scraping down the sides of the food processor with a rubber spatula as needed.

3. While continuing to pulse the food processor, gradually pour in the olive oil until you end up with a smooth paste.

4. Store pesto in an airtight container, covered with a thin layer of olive oil (about 1 tablespoon) to prevent oxidation, for up to 3 days.

VARIATION: Pesto is so versatile: Try spinach in place of the basil, and walnuts or pistachios instead of the pine nuts.

PER SERVING (1 TABLESPOON): Calories: 55; Total fat: 5.5g;
Total carbs: 0.5g; Fiber: 0g; Net carbs: 0.5g; Protein: 1g

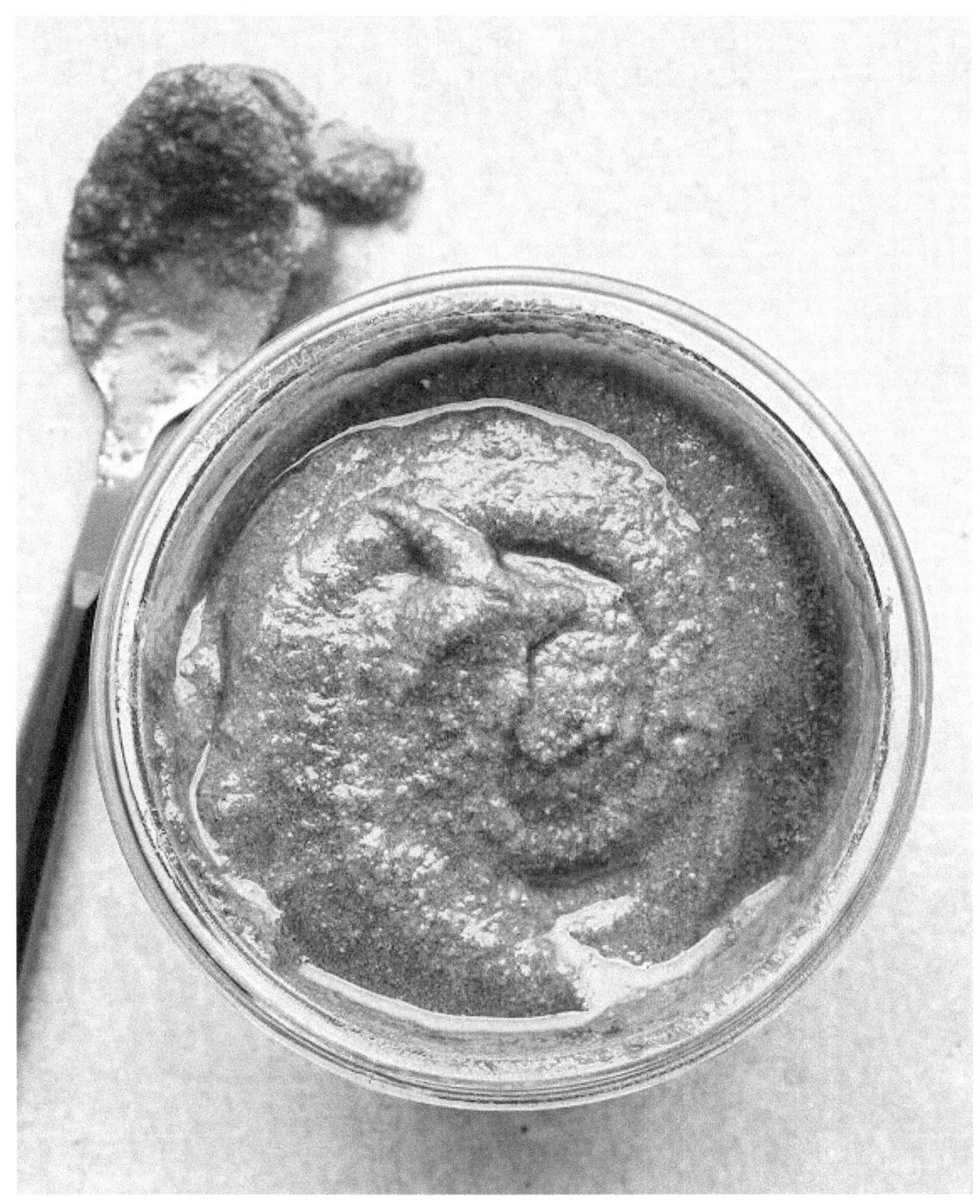

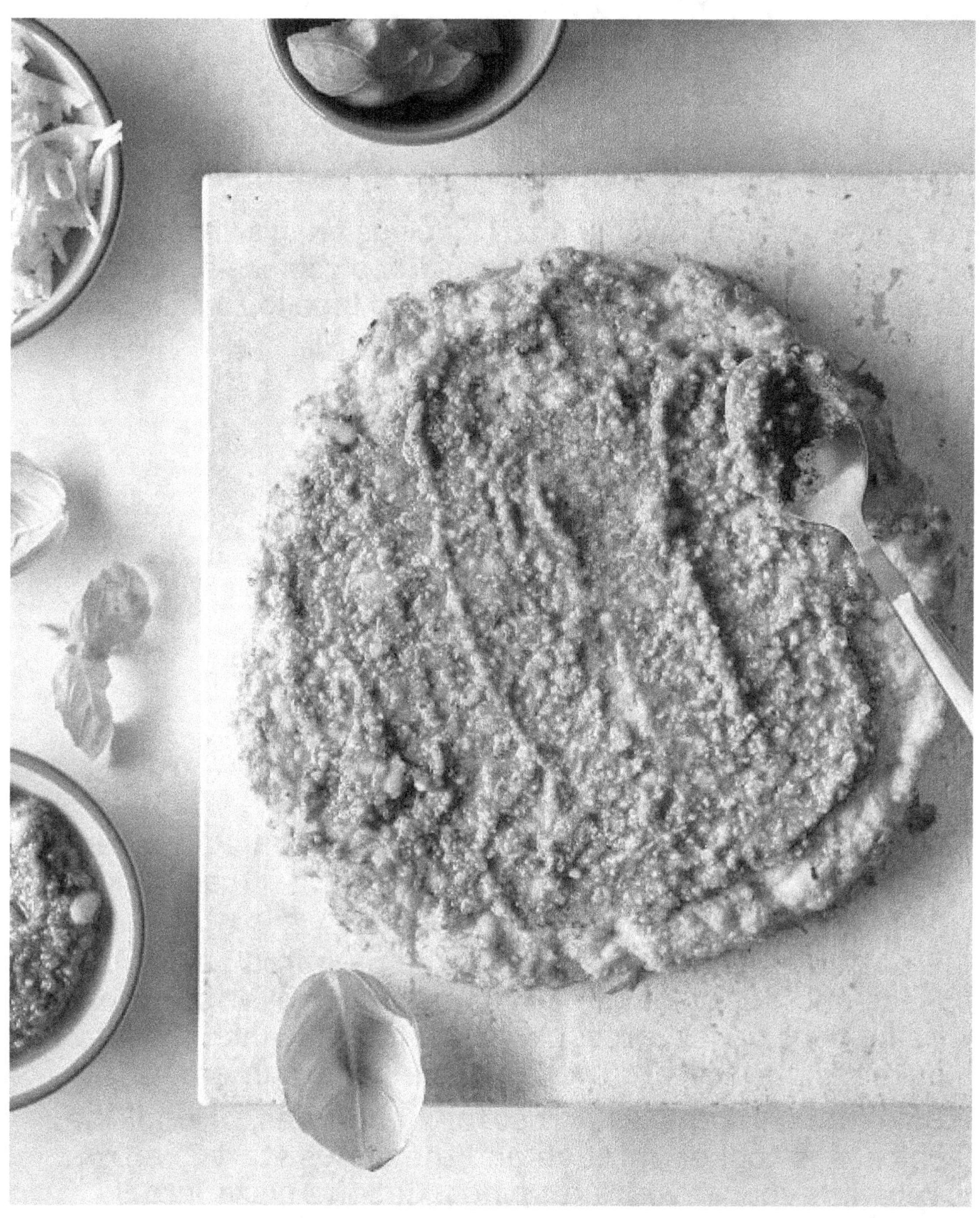

CHicken Pizza Crust

MAKES: **1 crust** | Quick Prep, Worth the Wait
PREP TIME: **10 minutes** | COOK TIME: **40 minutes**

You can enjoy your favorite pizza toppings on this keto-friendly pizza base made with ground chicken. For a caprese-style pizza, spread your chicken crust with <u>Pesto</u> and then top with sliced tomatoes, mozzarella cheese, and fresh basil.

1 pound ground chicken

¼ cup grated Parmesan cheese

½ cup shredded part-skim mozzarella cheese

½ teaspoon Italian seasoning

½ teaspoon garlic powder

½ teaspoon salt

½ teaspoon onion powder

¼ teaspoon red pepper flakes (optional)

1. Preheat the oven to 400°F. Line a baking sheet with parchment paper and set aside.

2. In a large bowl, combine the ground chicken, Parmesan, mozzarella, Italian seasoning, garlic powder, salt, onion powder, and red pepper flakes (if using). Mix well.

3. Transfer the chicken mixture to the prepared baking sheet. Place another piece of parchment paper over the mixture. Using your hands, press the meat into a ½-inch-thick circle or rectangle. Discard the top piece of parchment.

4. Bake the chicken pizza crust for 40 minutes, or until the chicken is cooked through and the edges start to brown. Top with your favorite toppings. Cut the pizza into 8 wedges.

5. Store any leftover crust in the refrigerator, covered, for up
   to 3 days.

INGREDIENT TIP: To make your own ground chicken, process 2
cups of cubed chicken breasts in a food processor until
smooth.

PER SERVING (1 WEDGE WITHOUT TOPPINGS): Calories: 110;
Total fat: 6g; Total carbs: 1g; Fiber: 0g; Net carbs: 1g; Protein:
13g

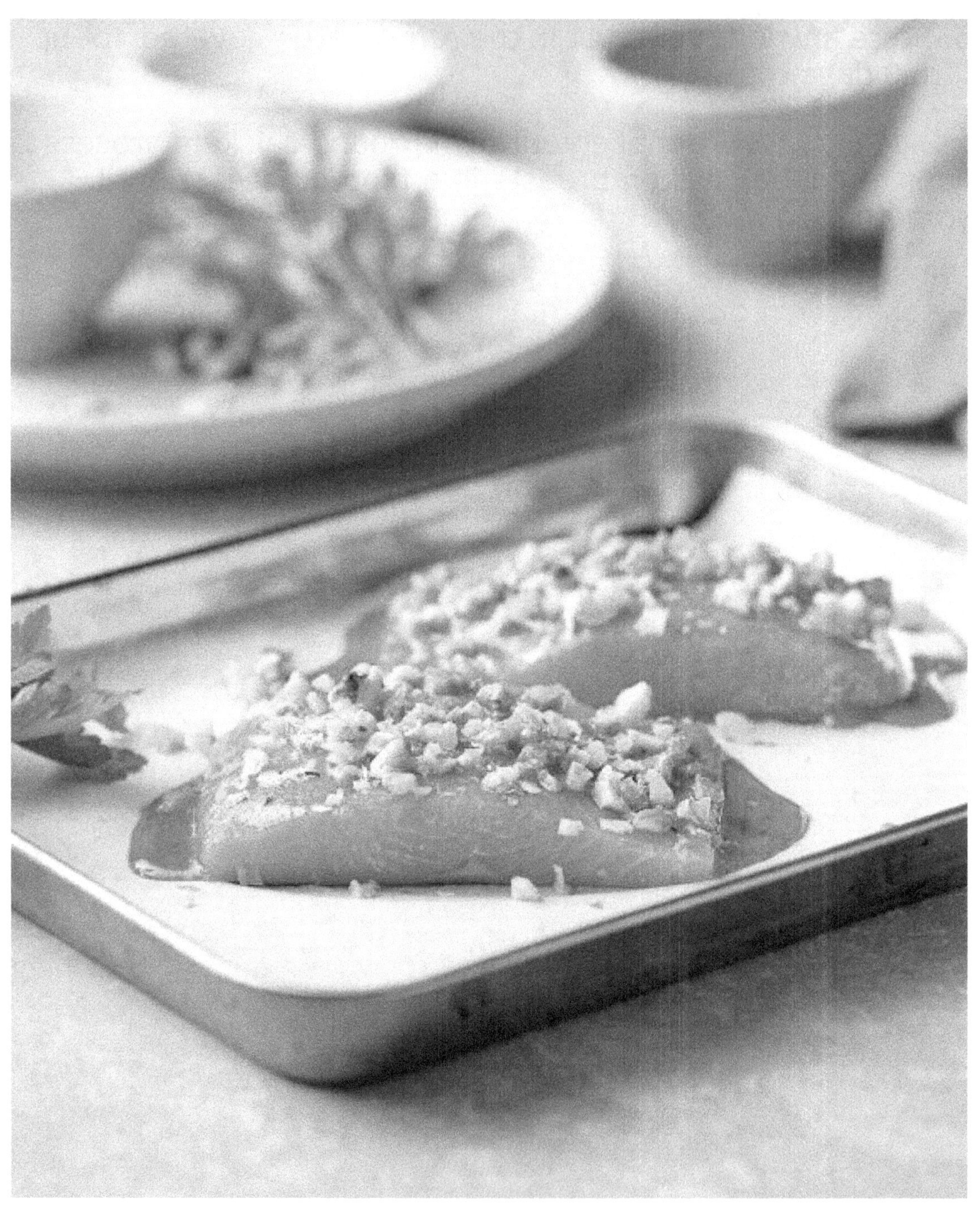

Measurement Conversions

VOLUME EQUIVALENTS	U.S. STANDARD	U.S. STANDARD (OUNCES)	METRIC (APPROXIMATE)
LIQUID	2 tablespoons	1 fl. oz.	30 mL
	¼ cup	2 fl. oz.	60 mL
	½ cup	4 fl. oz.	120 mL
	1 cup	8 fl. oz.	240 mL
	1½ cups	12 fl. oz.	355 mL
	2 cups or 1 pint	16 fl. oz.	475 mL
	4 cups or 1 quart	32 fl. oz.	1 L
	1 gallon	128 fl. oz.	4 L
DRY	⅛ teaspoon	—	0.5 mL
	¼ teaspoon	—	1 mL
	½ teaspoon	—	2 mL
	¾ teaspoon	—	4 mL
	1 teaspoon	—	5 mL
	1 tablespoon	—	15 mL
	¼ cup	—	59 mL
	⅓ cup	—	79 mL
	½ cup	—	118 mL
	⅔ cup	—	156 mL
	¾ cup	—	177 mL
	1 cup	—	235 mL
	2 cups or 1 pint	—	475 mL
	3 cups	—	700 mL
	4 cups or 1 quart	—	1 L
	½ gallon	—	2 L
	1 gallon	—	4 L

OVEN TEMPERATURES

FAHRENHEIT	CELSIUS (APPROXIMATE)
250°F	120°C
300°F	150°C
325°F	165°C
350°F	180°C
375°F	190°C
400°F	200°C
425°F	220°C
450°F	230°C

WEIGHT EQUIVALENTS

U.S. STANDARD	METRIC (APPROXIMATE)
½ ounce	15 g
1 ounce	30 g
2 ounces	60 g
4 ounces	115 g
8 ounces	225 g
12 ounces	340 g
16 ounces or 1 pound	455 g